ten minute
hips & thighs

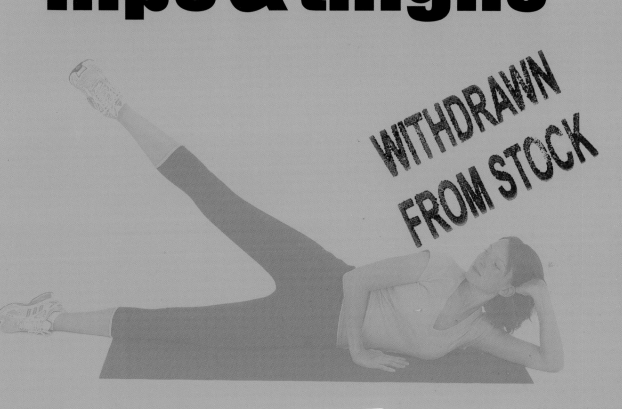

WITHDRAWN FROM STOCK

Chrissie Gallagher-Mundy

D1340725

ILLUSTRATED

Leabharlann Chontae Laoi

WITHDRAWN

Class No. 646.75

FROM STOCK

First published in the United Kingdom in 2003 by Cassell Illustrated,
a division of Octopus Publishing Group Limited
2–4 Heron Quays, London E14 4JP

Text copyright © Cassell Illustrated 2003
Design copyright © Cassell Illustrated 2003

The moral right of Chrissie Gallagher-Mundy to be identified as the author of
this work has been asserted in accordance with the Copyright, Designs and
Patents Act of 1988

All rights reserved. No part of this publication may be reproduced in any
material form (including photocopying or storing it in any medium by
electronic means and whether or not transiently or incidentally to some
other use of this publication) without the written permission of the copyright
owner, except in accordance with the provisions of the Copyright, Designs
and Patents Act 1988 or under the terms of a licence issued by the
Copyright Licensing Agency, 90 Tottenham Court Road, London W1P 9HE.
Applications for the copyright owner's written permission to reproduce any
part of this publication should be addressed to the publisher.

A CIP catalogue record for this book is available from the British Library

ISBN 1 84403 129 2

Produced and designed by SP Creative Design Ltd
Wickham Skeith, Suffolk, England
Editor: Heather Thomas
Designer: Rolando Ugolini
Special photography by Charlie Colmer
Models for photography: Emma Bradshaw and Ali Potter

Printed and bound in Hong Kong

**If you are pregnant or if you have a medical condition
that could be adversely affected by exercise or any doubts
about your health, consult a doctor before embarking on
any exercise programme.**

contents

using this
programme

This book provides a special programme of specific exercises that target your key problem areas – the hips and thighs. The exercises in the toning section are carefully calculated to cover the whole muscular area of these parts of the body. Too many people talk about hip exercises when really they are unclear where and what the muscles of the hips are. Many exercise manuals focus solely on the quadriceps muscles on the front of the thigh when there are other muscles on the upper leg to be considered, too. In this book, you will find precise information about the muscles you need to be working and how to exercise them most effectively.

In addition to the training exercises for key muscles, you will find some excellent cardiovascular (CV) workout suggestions. Working the cardiovascular system is important to your hip and thigh onslaught in three ways:

1 You need a strong heart and lungs to pump blood effectively to the muscles. Without this strong system, your body will not be able to build muscles as quickly as it should.

2 With constant cardio exercise, you will burn body fat – enabling you to reveal sleeker, stronger muscles as you build them.

3 Cardiovascular exercise gives you energy to feel a greater vitality and zest for life which will boost your life, as well as tone your hips and thighs!

Discover which muscles you need to exercise and how to work them most effectively.

Look at page 75 for a great cardiovascular and circulation-enhancing workout and try to do this routine at least twice per week. When you have built up your energy levels, throw in the interval training workout (see page 54) to really burn the calories and increase your fitness levels. If you can fit this routine in twice a week, you will start to notice an increase in your personal fitness. This will further tone your hips and thighs. Finally, try to perform the 10-minute focused toning on your hips and thighs three times per week. And don't forget your cool down at the end. Good luck!

Ideal timings

Rebounder workout	2 times weekly
Interval training	1-2 times weekly
Thigh toners	2 times weekly
Hip toners	2 times weekly

Suggested schedule

Rebounder + hip toners = 30 minutes
(Tuesday, Thursday and Friday)
Interval + thigh toners = 26 minutes
(Monday and Wednesday)

7

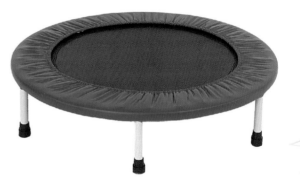

introduction

Our body shape is important to us. It contributes to the way in which we feel about ourselves – and how we feel about the world. So getting our bodies into optimum shape is something we would all like to be able to do. Well, the good news is that it is possible – and it need not take all day either!

With this 10-minute workout book you can make significant improvements in the shape and tone of your lower body, especially your hips and thighs, which will make you look and feel a whole lot fitter!

To look fit and well is important in the modern world so any body improvement manuals need to have this as the basis of their regime. This means that while you are working and challenging your body to make the muscles look leaner and the skin look firmer, you are also building greater strength and endurance for yourself. This, in turn, will give you more zest for life, more energy and a better-looking body in the process!

The hip and thigh area on a woman can be a notoriously difficult part of the body to keep sleek. Women are built to carry a certain amount of fat around this area. They tend to have larger hips than men and to gather greater fat stores in their hips and thighs during and after giving birth. Whilst it is a better place (medically speaking) to carry fat than around the abdomen (see page 14), many women find that this area becomes unsightly and difficult to keep firm and toned.

Our lower body should stay toned naturally – after all, we use our hips and thighs all the time as we walk around during the day. However, we also spend a lot of time sitting on our bottoms! This, together with the fact that we all have a tendency to eat more than we need, can encourage fat storage around this area. But don't worry – you can do something positive about the appearance of your hips and thighs and this book will show you how!

8

Hips and thighs can be a notoriously difficult part of the body to keep sleek but you can do something positive.

Your lower body should stay toned naturally – after all, you use your hips and thighs all the time as you walk around during the day. However, you also spend a lot of time sitting on your bottom!

Firstly, it will show you how to become more active – particularly with the lower body. It will also demonstrate how you can challenge the muscles of the lower body so that they get a perfectly aimed workout which leaves them strong and firm. Finally, you will find a portion of the workout that focuses on keeping the area supple and mobile so that all your lower body movements are executed safely. So why not get started now and follow the expert advice in this book and work on your hips and thighs intensely – you will be more than pleased with the results!

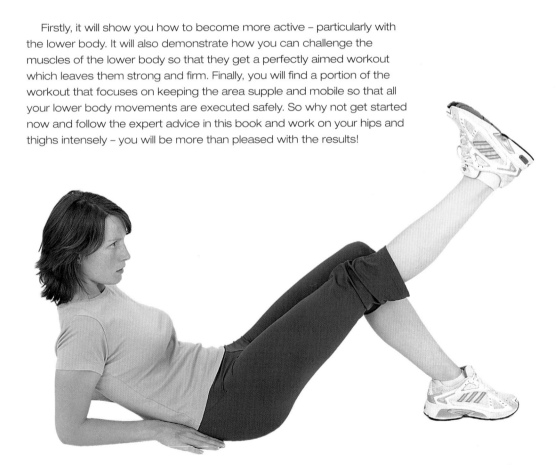

your body shape

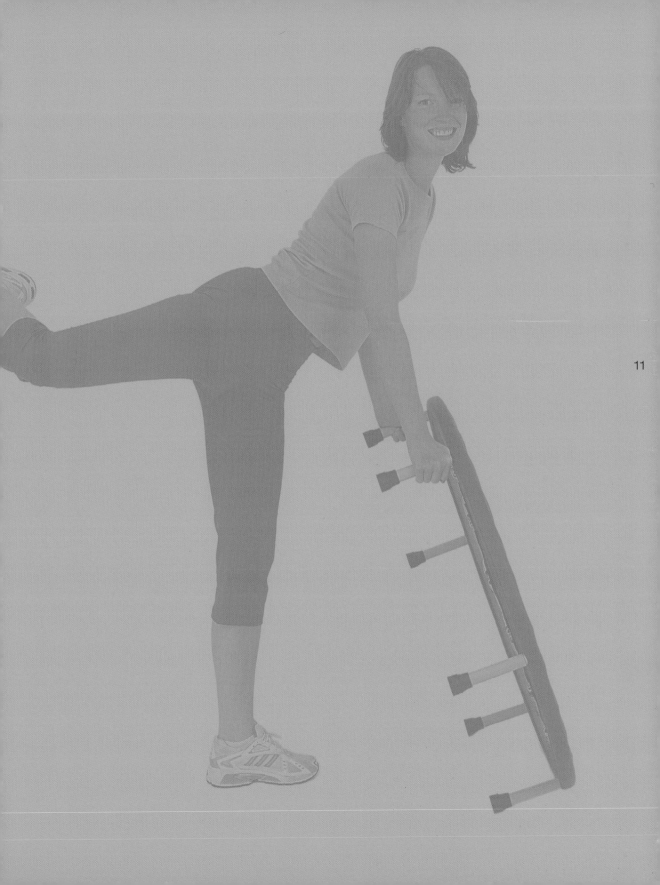

different body shapes

We all have different body shapes and, over the years, depending on their lifestyle and circumstances, some people can change their shape quite dramatically. Diets, sport and giving birth can all have an effect on our shape. Both men and women become concerned about some areas of the body more than others. The stomach – or the abdominals – is an area that most people need to work on in order to keep it well toned. For women particularly, it seems that the hips and thighs can also be difficult areas that are especially prone to problems. As women are designed to carry children, there is a tendency to lay down fat stores around these areas during pregnancy and they can be difficult to shift afterwards. Once new fat cells are created in the body they do not go away but wait to be filled! However, fat cells are not a problem unless you store unused calories. A healthy diet combined with exercise is all that's needed.

which shape are you?

It is generally accepted that there are three different body shapes. Some people refer to them as 'apple', 'pear' and 'stick' types. Apple types are generally large round the middle whereas pear types have larger hips and stick types tend to be straight.

Apple Shape

These people tend to store fat around the mid-section from the breasts to the hips. This will be true internally as well as externally, and therefore apple types are more at risk of diabetes, heart disease, stroke, high blood pressure and gall bladder disease. Apple types, however, can find it easy to lose weight if they really set their minds to it, and this will not only lower their health risk but also make a difference to how they look.

Pear Shape

Pear types tend to store fat around the hips and thighs and have hips that are wider than their shoulders. This means that their upper body can look disproportionately slim when compared to the bottom half. The risk of disease for pear types is lower than for apple shapes. However, in terms of how they look it can be frustratingly difficult for them to re-proportion their shape as when this type loses weight it tends to come off the upper body and not from the bottom half.

Stick Shape

Stick types tend to have a less obvious waist. They can be slim and trim yet look less curvaceous. Whilst they may not be overweight, their waist to hips ratio might be at the upper end of what is acceptable as their hips are smaller and their waist is larger than the classic frame. Stick types who put on too much weight tend to become more like apple types.

Health Risk Indicators

Body shape, however, is only one indicator of health risks. Others include:

- Heredity and family history
- Smoking and drinking levels
- Cholesterol levels
- Lifestyle habits such as exercise

Measure Yourself

You can measure your waist-hips ratio to see if you are an apple, pear or stick shape. Just do the following:

1 Measure your waist at the navel or just above – wherever you are smallest.

2 Measure your hips by bending the knees and pressing the thighs outwards. Measure around where the hip bones are.

3 Divide your waist size by your hip size to get the ratio. Women should have a ratio of 0.8 or less; men should have 0.95 or less.

- If you have apple type tendencies you need to plan a programme of healthy living (and weight loss if necessary) to combat any of the risk factors to your health that you may have.
- If you are a pear type you have less health risks, which is good news! However you will need to focus your fitness training to move as much excess fat as possible from your lower body.
- If you are a stick type you may have to work harder to define your waist. Keep your torso twisting and bending throughout your life to stay defined in this area.

Which shape are you – apple, pear or stick shape?

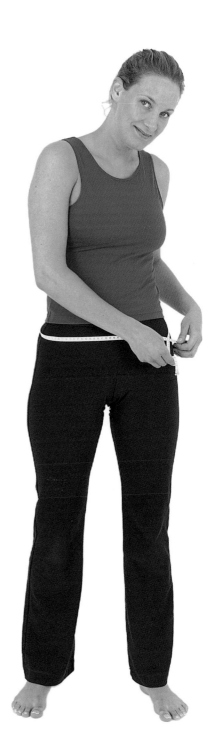

15

heavy hips and thighs

The problem with a thicker lower body is that the fat can be difficult to shift. Even though the health risks are better for a pear shape this isn't much consolation if you can't wear the outfits you want or you have trouble buying dresses that end up being too loose on your top half and too tight on your larger lower half! Unfortunately, there are no miracle exercises that will shrink your lower half and suddenly make you completely in proportion. Some people (and this might be you) have larger pelvises and hip bones so that no amount of exercise or lifestyle changes will alter your basic bone structure. The good news, however, is you can make the best of what you have!

Perception

First of all, think positive and remember that while there are pear and apple types there are also many other shapes and none of them are wrong! There is another classification of body types called somatotyping where the body is defined in terms of its musculature and fat tendencies. Indeed, there are now some studies that talk of defining the body into over 40 different types to make the point that tall, slim shapes are not the only healthy shapes. The somatotypes, however, are useful in helping you to understand how your body works and thereby how you might approach your training programme.

Ectomorph Shape

This is the long, tall body shape that you tend to see in catwalk models, ballet dancers and long-distance runners. These people tend to have difficulty in gaining weight or large muscle masses, no matter how hard they train. Only a small proportion of the population has this type of body.

Mesomorph Shape

Mesomorphs gain muscle quickly and tend to have slightly stockier builds with shorter arms and legs. They are strong although they may find it more difficult to lose weight and may weigh in heavier on the scales because of their higher muscle to fat ratio.

Endomorph Shape

These types tend to have a higher body fat percentage and have a harder time losing body fat, even when they diet and exercise. They may have softer, less muscular frames and are well built for endurance events.

Your Type

You may well be a combination of all these types or you may be able to recognize in yourself one particular type that seems most like you. The thing to remember, with regard to these categories, is to accept what you are and train in harmony with your type.

For instance, if you have heavier hips and thighs the chances are you will be an endomorph (or have strong elements of this). If you are an endomorph you need to work at building muscle and keeping existing muscle firm and toned. Although you may not be attracted to muscle-building-type workouts, these are important for you – as they are for the ectomorph.

Ectomorphs tend to be attracted to long-distance running and other cardiovascular regimes and, again, may well shy away, by choice, from muscle-building regimes.

Mesomorphs are the opposite. Resistance work comes easy to them and they are often far more inclined to opt for this kind of fitness training or sport than for cardiovascular training.

The thing to remember, with regard to these categories, is to accept what you are and train in harmony with your type.

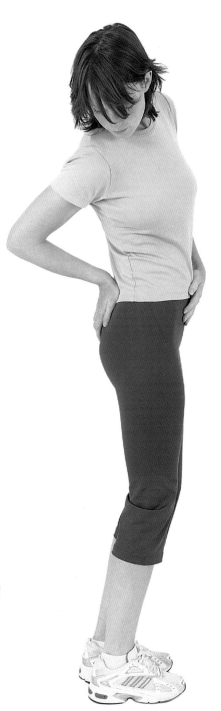

your best shape

To get your best shape possible, you need to remember the following: whatever your type (see page 14) you need to keep your body fit and flexible for as much of your life as you can. But how do you stay fit and what does being fit mean? To be really fit you need to do the following exercise.

Muscle Resistance Exercise

You should give your body regular muscle resistance exercise. Working muscles against resistance strengthens them and makes them more capable of lifting and pulling heavier loads. If you can lift and pull effectively you can perform everyday (and non-everyday) jobs without risk of injury or aches and pains. As you work your muscles they pull on the bones, stimulating bone growth and slowing down bone loss. This reduces your risk of osteoporosis as you age, where the bones thin and can fracture.

Cardiovascular Exercise

You should give your body regular cardiovascular exercise so that the heart and lungs are being challenged regularly. When you do this the heart muscle stays strong and the lungs work efficiently. This means your body can use fat stores efficiently for energy. If your heart and lungs are working well, you will be able to keep going (at almost anything) and cope better with the many demands in your day. People who have good fit cardiovascular systems will feel more energetic and full of life than those who do not.

Stretching Exercise

You should give your body a regular stretching session. Muscles move us by contraction and those contractions need to be stretched out from time to time to keep our full range of movement available. Many people assume that as we get older we lose flexibility naturally. Therefore we assume that loss of range of movement and being able to do the tasks we could do as a child is normal. In fact, many studies indicate that most of the lowering of physical performance as we age is down to lack of use as opposed to lack of potential. As we age, we sit around more and become less energetic. If you fail to challenge your muscles, they simply decline and atrophy (waste away) due to lack of use. In the same way, muscles become shortened and less pliable if they are not stretched and stressed regularly.

By keeping your muscles and your bones stimulated and moving them around, you not only warm the synovial fluid between the joints but also encourage mobility and smooth, flowing movement. If you have this ability at your disposal then you can perform everyday movements and intense sporting movement with agility and balance. Your co-ordination will be better and your mind-body paths will be practised. In this way, you will have improved balance and control of your body, which helps to prevent injuries and allows you to move more gracefully with ease and confidence.

19

weight loss

Losing weight is a difficult thing to do! Too many times, extra fat on our bodies seems to creep up on us and, without us realizing it, we feel that in an instant we have gained two kilos (five pounds)! Then it seems to take forever to lose that weight – with days and weeks of hard slog to shed what seemed to come on in a moment! No wonder there is that phrase: 'a moment in the mouth – a month on the hips!' This perception, however, is mistaken. Weight gain and weight loss happen in the same way – gradually. As the calories we consume in the form of food exceed the energy demands of our bodies, then the excess is stored in fat cells under the skin. Conversely, in the opposite scenario, if we are more active than the amount of calories we have consumed, then the fat cells become depleted as we use them up to meet our body's energy needs.

The rate at which we use up energy depends on our individual make-up and metabolism. As with body types (see page 14), some people find it easier to lose and gain weight than others. Regardless of your inherited and non-hereditary characteristics, however, there are some basic guidelines that anyone can follow to aid and speed up their weight loss.

Be Active

The less you do, the less food you need, so the easiest way to gain weight is to sit around a lot and eat a lot. If you are trying to lose weight, then reverse this! Take a long, hard look at your week and see how active you really are. Look at your lifestyle and see if you can replace some of your TV watching time with activity. Instead of taking the car everywhere, could you try walking? These little changes can make a big difference over the weeks and months.

Cut Down on Alcohol

Try not to drink too much alcohol; it really does get easily stored as fat. Again, cutting back on even one glass a week can make a big difference to how you look at the end of three months!

Keep Your Diet Realistic

There are weird and wonderful diets out there but the best is the one you can stick to month in and month out. This is called the 'sensible eating' diet. Diets that advocate cutting away one-third of your eating choice, as in 'cut out carbs' or 'cut out fat', are hard to follow and unsociable to stick to long term. The key is to eat a varied diet and not to over-eat.

Eat Regularly

This keeps your blood sugar at a happy level (for you and others). Starving yourself will slow down your metabolism and may even lead to out-of-control over-eating at some point.

Be Realistic

There are so many diets out there offering instant results so try to be realistic about your weight loss goals. You must be patient and stick at the diet you have chosen even if it takes time. Gradual, steady weight loss is preferable to a quick fix. Remember that just cutting out an extra glass of wine or doing an additional five-minute stretching session will help to tip the balance over a period of three months.

If you lose one kilo (two pounds) a month, you are doing well!

your **hip** muscles

Before you can really begin to shape and tone your hips, you need to know where and what the muscles are around this area! There is no one muscle that constitutes the hip. When most people commonly refer to the hips they are talking about the hip bones which are the top part of the pelvis. The pelvis is bone and therefore cannot be toned or altered in any real way. However, there are surrounding muscles that make up what we think of as the hip area, and it's good to have a clear picture of where the muscles are and how to work them effectively. There are three groups of muscle that pass over the hip joint. They are as follows:

- The buttock muscles
- The groin muscles
- The hip flexors

If you are to keep the hip area as toned and shaped as you like, you need to make sure that all three of these muscles groups are strong.

The Buttock Muscles

The buttock muscles are also a group of three. They are as follows:

- The gluteus maximus
- The gluteus minimus
- The gluteus medius

These muscles stabilize the hip joint when you are putting your body weight on one foot and are particularly stressed, e.g. when you run up a hill. The large gluteus maximus is responsible for the powerful backward drive of the leg whereas the medius and minimus stabilize the hip as you run down.

The Groin Muscles

The groin muscles are as follows:

- The adductor muscles (long and short)

These muscles originate from the pubic bone and attach to the upper part of the thigh bone (femur). They work powerfully when running; swinging the legs forwards and rotating them outwards in relation to the hips. Strengthening and lengthening them will shape the thigh and guard against groin injuries.

The Hip Flexors

The hip flexor muscles are as follows:

- Iliacus
- Psoas muscle
- Together called the iliopsoas

Allowing powerful flexion at the hip joint, these are toned in such everyday activities as walking, running and stair climbing. You need strong abdominal muscles to hold the lumbar spine in place when the iliopsoas is under stress.

your thigh muscles

The muscles of the thigh are technically the ones that work the knee joint. Again, there are three main types of muscle, which are as follows:

The Quadriceps Femoris

This is the group name for the muscles that run along the front of the thigh. It is made up of the following muscles:

- The rectus femoris
- The vastus intermedius
- The vastus lateralis
- The vastus medius

The rectus femoris crosses the hip joint and acts as a hip flexor. The other muscles are responsible for extending the knee and stabilizing the knee cap. Moves that involve bending – correctly – and pushing straight will all help to strengthen the thigh muscles.

The Hamstrings

The muscles that flex the knee joint are the group commonly known as the hamstrings. They are made up as follows:

- The biceps femoris
- The semi membranosus
- The semi tendinosus

These muscles run along the back of the thigh. The biceps femoris can rotate the lower leg so that the foot points outwards. The hamstring muscles generally stay relatively well toned but you can do specific exercises to strengthen them further. It is also important to keep these muscles flexible. Stretching them out after frequent contractions is essential (see page 117). To shape and sculpt your thighs, you need to strengthen and stretch them, back and front.

Other Thigh Muscles

There are two other muscles in the thigh of which you should be aware. They are as follows:

- The sartorius muscle
- The gracilis muscle

The sartorius muscle starts at the outside of the pelvis and extends down to the inner side of the knee. It is the longest muscle in the body and has many functions, particularly when bending and opening out the leg, e.g. when you sit cross-legged. It is sometimes referred to as the tailor's muscle. The gracilis muscle runs along the inner thigh. It aids movement such as bending the knees and pulling the leg in toward the centre. Both muscles will benefit from the hip and thigh exercises in this book.

active quiz

Do this quiz to discover where and how you can change your behaviour. Just answer the questions opposite honestly and then turn over the page to see how you have scored. There are no right or wrong answers for this quiz. The results are not high or low scores but simply things for you to think about which may prompt ideas. As you answer the questions, you may start examining how you manage your life and spend your time and also how much activity and exercise you could fit in.

1 I play sport

a   More than six times per month

b   Once a week or less

c   Once a month

2 I put aside time for formal exercise

a   Three times a week

b   Once a week

c   Once a month

3 I over-eat

a   Never

b   Sometimes

c   Frequently

4 I drink alcohol

a   Two or less glasses a couple of nights a week

b   Two or less glasses most nights

c   More than two glasses most nights

5 I do five minutes of limbering/stretching

a   Every few days

b   Once a week

c   Once a month

6 I play active games with my children

a   Weekly

b   Monthly

c   Yearly

7 I have gaps between formal exercise of

a   1–3 days

b   1–3 weeks

c   1–3 months

8 I read up on health and fitness

a   Weekly

b   Monthly

c   Yearly

9 I watch TV for three hours solid

a   Several times a month

b   Several times a week

c   Most evenings

learn from your answers

Question 1

If you answered: **a** Well done, keep it up!

b Once a week is OK if you're doing other activities too. If you are playing a tough sport only once a week you need to be doing some conditioning for it too.

c Take up a sport or an activity that you do more frequently; decide on something and put it in your diary now!

Question 2

If you answered: **a** Well done, keep it up!

b If you're not doing a sport as well, you need to do more formal exercise. Once a week is not enough if you want to stay fit and un-fat for the next 20 years.

c Find six slots a month for yourself to do exercise. Join a gym or simply get yourself a home programme – but you need to do something to keep those hips and thighs in shape long term!

Question 3

If you answered: **a** Sounds like portion control isn't a big issue for you – that's lucky!

b Drink water frequently – this will help you feel fuller and eat slowly. Try to register when you don't feel hungry any more and stop at that point.

c One of the best ways to stop over-eating is before you take a second helping wait 20 minutes. In that time your stomach will register you are full.

Question 4

If you answered: **a** One glass of red wine per night is thought of as beneficial. No more though!

b Have at least one alcohol-free day. One glass, rather than two, will keep the calories under control for those slim hips and thighs!

c More than two glasses most nights is too many calories for your thighs and too much alcohol for your liver. Have at least one alcohol-free day.

Question 5

If you answered: **a** This is good. It will keep you feeling supple and flexible.

b Twice or three times a week will keep you feeling much more supple.

c Stretching and limbering, particularly in the legs, are important and especially as we get older. Install a programme (it doesn't have to be very long) of stretching now!

Question 6

If you answered: **a** This is good. All activity will help you stay fit and it will set a good example for your children, too.

b Find more active things for you and your family to do. Plan an activity twice a month.

c What about walks in the park? Bike riding? Skipping outdoors? There are many active things you can do with younger people to keep them happy and you fit!

Question 7

If you answered: **a** Well done, keep it up!

b Don't allow such long gaps between exercising, especially if you are trying to lose weight.

c You need to exercise more regularly than this – otherwise, your muscles will decrease and you will be less strong. You may also find it tougher to lose weight.

Question 8

If you answered: **a** Well done, keep it up!

b The more you read, the more you will be inspired to keep up your fitness so read more.

c Try to read up on health and fitness; it will inspire you to make small changes that can get big results!

Question 9

If you answered: **a** TV's OK but stretch when the adverts come on!

b Could you bear to switch the TV off for just 45 minutes on one of those nights? And do the 10-minute workout instead!

c Lose one night per week's TV watching and do some exercise instead.

great-looking
hips and thighs

Looking and feeling
your best is down to
two things: diet and
exercise. If you
have excess fat on
your bottom half, then you
need to lose some body
fat. And if your muscles
are untoned and flabby,
then you need to do
some serious exercise.
Your best bet is to do
both! If you take this
two-pronged attack to
your hips and thighs
they will improve
within two months.

Get Your Eating Habits in Order

Follow some basic guidelines for eating and they should help to keep your calorie consumption in check. It is so much easier to over-eat nowadays. There is a plethora of gorgeous-tasting food around – readily available – so we need to develop some strategies for not over-indulging all the time.

Get Leaner Without Taking Food Away!

● Drink water regularly. The amount recommended is 6–8 good-sized glasses per day. This will help give the body what it needs and stop you getting dehydrated, which would lower you energy levels. If you drink regularly, you may also find you are less hungry which will help you to resist that calorie overload.

● As a general rule, choose foods that are lower in fat and higher in fibre.

● Try to add things to your plate rather than take them away! Too many people perceive diets as starvation. Indeed, some are, but the best way is to make sure you are getting the vitamins and minerals you need. Make sure at every meal you have at least one fruit or vegetable on your plate. With larger meals you should have two.

● Therefore at breakfast, for example, if all you normally eat is a bowl of cereal you need to add a fruit, perhaps some berries or a sliced banana. If your breakfast is toast with a small scraping of butter and some spread, add a fruit to this too – a banana or even a peeled and sliced apple. If you are someone who can't face something so large in the morning and usually just gets by on a cup of coffee, then try squeezing some fruits to make a juice cocktail or grab the blender and add some milk or yogurt to the juice to make a nutrient-packed milkshake. Smoothies are very popular so why not experiment with different fruits and flavours?

● What is your average lunch? If it is a sandwich, then add another layer to it! Add some extra tomato, ask the vendor for extra salad or buy an extra avocado to go with it.

● At dinnertime make sure your plate has two vegetables on it. Or even three! Always try to have two different vegetables that go alongside any proteins or fats on your plate. The brighter the colours of the vegetables the more vitamins you are packing in. For dessert, even if you have a portion of chocolate cake, add some fruit alongside: a slice of pineapple perhaps or some fresh peach along with your ice cream. An afternoon cake? Add some banana to it!

29

Reduce Your Calorie Intake

The purpose of this adding policy is simple. As you add more to your plate, you won't feel as though you are starving yourself. You will also be getting the high-quality vitamins and minerals that your body needs. It is currently recommended that everybody should eat five fruit/vegetable portions per day to guard against disease and keep us in optimum health. Not only this, but as you fill your plate with fruit and vegetables there will be less room on it for the other stuff! In this way, without too much hardship, you will be cutting calories. If you reduce your calorie intake, you will lose fat.

Get your Exercise Regime in Place

Exercise does so much for the body that it is amazing that more people don't do it! In general terms, it has the following functions:

- Exercise will tone the muscles of the body, helping to keep them healthy and strong and ready for action.
- As you move and work against resistance you pull on the muscles, which, in turn, pull on the bones keeping them strong and stimulated. This can help slow down diseases such as osteoporosis.

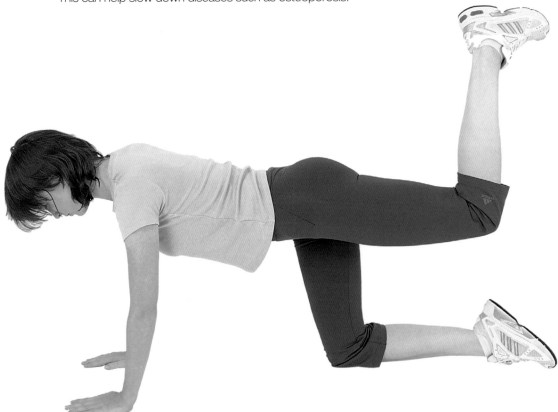

Exercise uses a lot of energy and calories. As you work out and use up extra calories, your body shape will get firmer.

- Exercise helps release endorphins into the blood stream, which give you a feeling of well being. Therefore stress reduction and relaxation can be gained from regular exercise.
- Exercise, particularly cardiovascular work, strengthens the heart muscle and works out the lungs, giving you better stamina and endurance and more energy for your everyday activities. This can also help guard against all manner of diseases.
- Regular activity will keep your brain to muscle links working, making you more co-ordinated, more in control of your body and less likely to injure it.

Specific Hip and Thigh Exercise

Exercise, formal or otherwise, uses up significant amounts of energy and calories. Therefore as you work out and use up extra calories (that you weren't using before) you will start to deplete your fat stores and lose fat around your hips and thighs.

Certain exercise regimes focus on the lower body (see page 50 on walking) and this will help tone and lose fat from these areas. Although spot toning alone doesn't work, you do need to do exercises that tone and shape the offending area. As you lose body fat you will need to work on the hip and thigh muscles to get them in shape. Some of the muscles of the hip and thigh area – for example, the buttock muscle at the back of the hips and the quadriceps muscle group at the front of the thighs – are large muscles. They will look great when they are shaped and sculpted!

As you focus on this area you can learn how to use the lower body more effectively and improve the flexibility and mobility in the joints around this area.

part

2

ways to boost your circulation

32

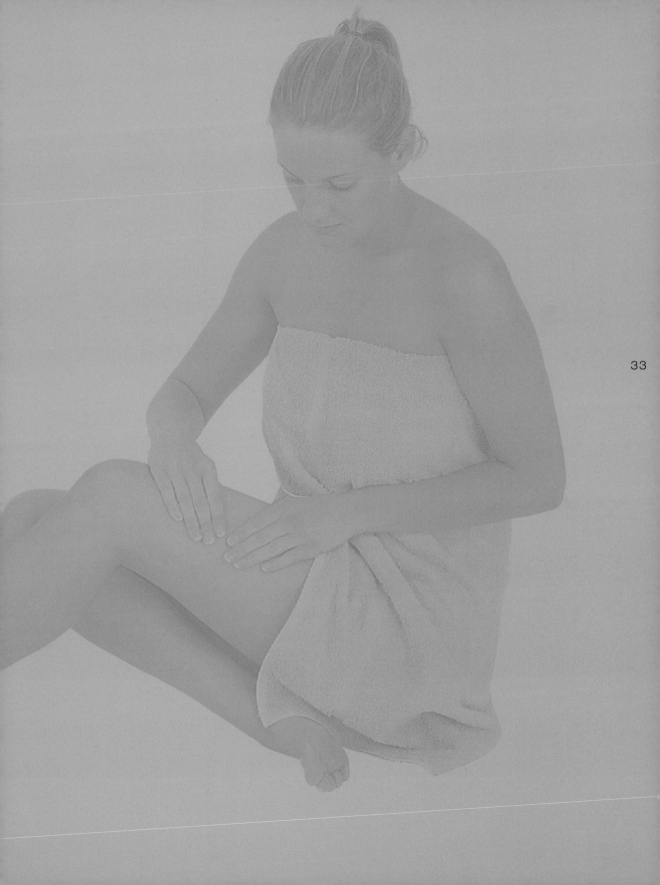

the truth about

There has long been a great debate about cellulite. What is it and does it really exist? And if you have it, what is the best way to get rid of it? The real answer, which you will not find in any women's magazines, is this: you cannot get rid of cellulite.

You need it! You can, however, improve the look of your body, cellulite and all! Do you want to know what cellulite really is? It is fat – FAT. Plain and simple. Pure and simple. This is not the answer you want to hear, is it? You would prefer it to be the result of

cellulite

something in the water you drink, perhaps a condition you can catch from someone else, or something that can be massaged away, just as it arrived when you weren't massaging yourself enough. You would probably prefer to talk to Dr X. Did you see his programme on television? He is the fat person's guardian angel. He is desperately trying to verify his claim that fatness is a virus which spreads and can be caught and, at some stage presumably, cured. But it won't happen, not that way.

35

fat or toxins?

Fat (cellulite) is, simply, the storage of excess food. The food you eat is converted into energy to be transported around the body. Thus, the body breaks down the food that goes into your stomach and turns it into energy ready for the muscles to utilize, then stores the rest. What most people mean when they refer to cellulite is the fat stores that are visible beneath the skin. And hey – get real here – we've all got them!

In a study of 1,000 women of all shapes and sizes from all the different continents, Dr Len Kravitz (Doctor of Exercise Science at the University of New Mexico) observed that all the women studied had cellulite!

Basically, cellulite is fat – no more, no less – but the way in which the fat is stored can appear more unsightly on some people than on others. It is stored in the subcutaneous layer of the skin and held in place by constricting bands of connective tissue. As we age and the skin thins, or as we fill out our fat cells, this connective tissue and fat cell network can become more visible, resulting in the tell-tale orange-peel-type skin we associate with cellulite. It is a bit like saying we all have teeth; it's just that some people's teeth are better looking than others! Now there is the crux of the matter. Who has got the best-looking cellulite?

Of course, men also store fat but they store it deeper in the skin than women and tend to amass it around their mid section. However, the good news for women is that it is safer to carry fat on your thighs than on your stomach where fat gets into the blood stream faster. And you can do some positive things to help attack that cellulite and improve its appearance.

Don't panic – this book will help bust your cellulite blues in the most practical and healthy way possible.

Don't be Distracted

As humans, we all evolved in the same way and are all built to survive. Being able to store fat is one of our keenest survival mechanisms. Women's bodies are designed to store more fat than mens. This is because we need to have enough energy stored to give birth and feed our offspring afterwards. Men do store fat – some men even have cellulite – and some sport spare tyres. It is all excess storage. The fact is that some people look better with it than others and, in the right light, you would hardly know it was there. The reason why I am labouring this point is that, in your quest to look your best, you can throw away any unhelpful theories that will simply distract you from the real task in hand. Getting yourself toned and fit will reduce the appearance of the fat that you are carrying.

Because it has become so important to look slim and fat free (the opposite of earlier centuries), there are endless remedies and urban myths that surround fat loss and cellulite. Companies talk about fat-burning pills, thigh-reducing creams and vague hormones and toxins, which supposedly add to your fat stores (cellulite). Don't believe any of it! There may come a day when someone does invent a fat-reducing pill (and if so, they will be a zillionaire overnight) or, more likely, an appetite suppressant pill, but so far this has not happened and it is very unlikely to happen in the near future.

So you can only work with the information we know to be true today – and until a miracle cure for eating too much comes along – you will just have to work with the following established facts.

Fact 1

The excess calories you consume are stored as fat. The more fat you have, the more it will show. It might show as an increase in size or as an orange peel appearance under your skin. So reducing your fat stores will help.

Fact 2

Toned lean muscle fills out the skin and keeps the connective tissue which holds the fat cells taut. Therefore toned muscle will help improve the appearance of any fat that you are carrying.

Fact 3

As Wayne L. Westcott, PhD of UK Wellness. points out: "Cellulite is not a cosmetic problem and so cannot be cured by cosmetic solutions."

there is a place for massage

Whilst massage is not a cure for carrying too much fat, it can help you in your quest for good-looking hips and thighs. Aiding the body's own natural cleansing systems can only improve the appearance of both the skin and muscle tissue in these areas. There have been numerous studies which show that massage can help:

- Improve the circulation and movement of lymph fluids
- Enhance and nourish the skin
- Promote deeper and easier breathing benefiting the whole system
- Relieve muscle tension and stiffness

The main techniques that your massage therapist might use for improving the hip and thigh area are explained below. Although you may like to try some of these basic techniques on yourself, you will gain far more if you can find a friend or partner to do it for you! This enables you to relax fully and absorb the benefits! See page 42 for self-massage techniques with a skin brush.

Effleurage

This is the technique of long, sliding strokes that therapists use in the first stages of a massage. They use the whole of their hands and the pads of the thumbs. When massaging the limbs, all strokes should be directed towards the heart to spur on the blood and lymphatic flow.

Petrissage

This is where the therapist begins to lift the muscles up and away from the bones. Some rolling and squeezing movements may be employed with a gentle pressure to aid the circulation. This boosted circulation helps to clear toxins from the muscles and nerve tissue.

Tapotement

For this technique, the therapist uses briskly and firmly applied percussive movements, using the hands to strike or tap for invigoration. This can be done with the edge of the hands, the tips of the fingers or even with a closed fist. Tapotement stimulates the muscles and releases tension; it also helps to prevent muscle spasms and alerts the individual being massaged.

skin brushing

Skin brushing has long been considered an effective tool for making your hip and thigh area look as good as possible. Although it will not melt away fat, it can help boost the circulation and, thereby, the appearance of the overall area. If the skin on your hips, bottom or thighs is not as smooth as it should be, if you have unsightly pimples under the skin or other clogged pores, skin brushing can really even out skin tone.

How It Works

Skin brushing means what it says: it is the action of taking a bristled brush and sweeping it along the surface of the skin. The skin is an organ – like other organs of the body – and it is constantly replenishing itself as the old skin is replaced with new. Skin brushing will slough off the dead skin cells and rid you of the sweat and other surface minerals that have come up through the skin. It is done with a dry, stiff-bristled brush which grips onto the skin a little as you brush and thus really boosts the lymphatic flow under the skin. For circulation and lymphatic boosting purposes, skin brushing is great as a precursor to massage, which then works deeper on the muscle tissue. It is also an easier beauty routine to carry out on yourself than massage, which is more effective when done by someone else.

How to Get Started

First assemble your tools! You need a large, oval-shaped stiff-bristled brush. Do not wet it as wet brushing is not as effective for circulation boosting. Seat yourself comfortably in a warm room with a towel beneath your feet and some oil handy for afterwards.

- A brush with a removable handle is a good idea as the handle is useful for reaching behind you and you can then remove the handle when you brush the skin at the front. (This presumes that eventually you will perform a whole body brushing routine.)
- Perform your skin brushing routine before you have a bath or shower.
- Starting at the knees, make long, large sweeps up the side of one leg, then up the front and along the inside of the leg, then finally around the back of the thigh.

For circulation and lymphatic boosting purposes, skin brushing is a great precursor to massage.

The quality and general appearance of the skin should improve as you encourage the skin to rejuvenate.

The Benefits

You should notice an increased circulation to the brushed areas of the thighs with clearer, firmer skin.

- The skin around the thighs (where many women pack fat) can become quite pale, and cold-skin brushing will make the skin warmer and pinker as you bring blood to the area.
- Aim to brush once a day all over the thighs for 5–6 minutes. Within two weeks, you should notice the skin buffing up and shining and its texture and appearance will improve.
- If you suffer from any kind of swelling or oedema around the thighs or ankles, you may well find that skin brushing will help to reduce puffiness and water retention. This can be particularly beneficial during menstruation as you can still skin brush at this time.
- The quality and general appearance of the skin should improve as you encourage the skin to rejuvenate.

What to Do Afterwards

After your skin brushing session, take a bath with some moisturizer in it and relax. Feel the tingling sensation you have created and breathe deeply. Drink a glass of water as you soak. When you get out of the bath, give the whole body a brisk rub down and apply some oil to the brushed areas.

- Aromatherapy oils can be used in skin brushing. Essential lavender oil is particularly good for the circulation.
- Other oils, such as chamomile, geranium or rosemary, *may* also be appropriate but you will need to check which is the best oil for you to use with a qualified aromatherapist first.
- Skin brushing is a good idea if you plan to use fake tan on your hips and thighs. It will really exfoliate your skin, brushing away any dead skin cells and making it as smooth as possible for the tan base.

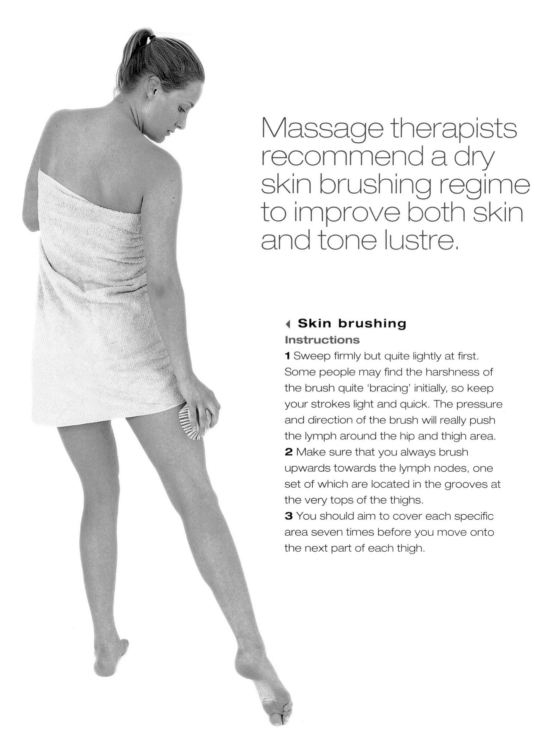

Massage therapists recommend a dry skin brushing regime to improve both skin and tone lustre.

42

◀ **Skin brushing**

Instructions

1 Sweep firmly but quite lightly at first. Some people may find the harshness of the brush quite 'bracing' initially, so keep your strokes light and quick. The pressure and direction of the brush will really push the lymph around the hip and thigh area.

2 Make sure that you always brush upwards towards the lymph nodes, one set of which are located in the grooves at the very tops of the thighs.

3 You should aim to cover each specific area seven times before you move onto the next part of each thigh.

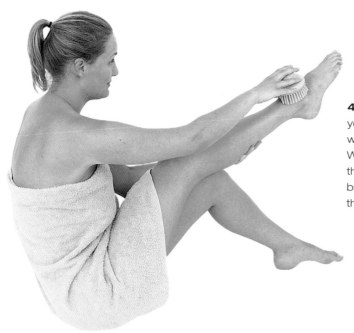

4 Once you have brushed both thighs, you may like to start at your feet and work upwards stroking along the calves. When you brush your feet, you will notice the dead skin cells falling away as you brush. You may also want to brush over the top of the thighs onto the buttocks.

5 As you brush regularly, your skin will become more accustomed to the sensation and will not be as sensitive as when you began. You may notice also that some areas of your skin are more sensitive than others.

6 Do not brush over any areas of skin that are cut or raw and, likewise, avoid areas with eczema or psoriasis.

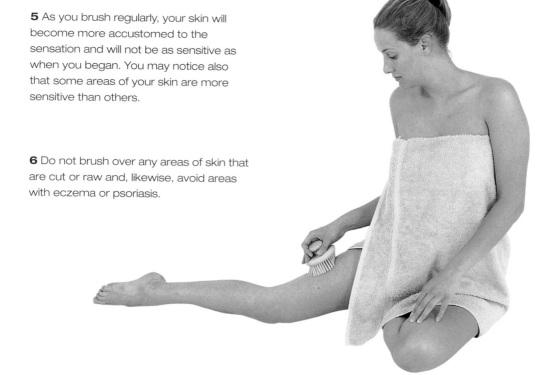

boost your energy

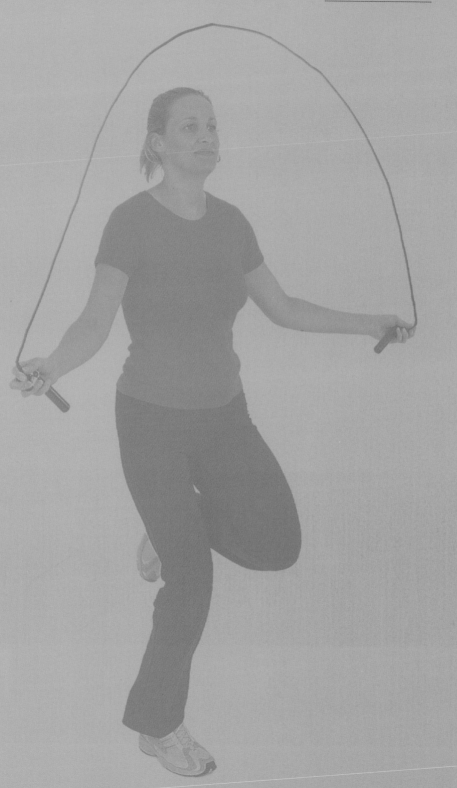

the importance

There are now many different sports and activities that are available out in the great wide world and you may be wondering which are best for you when you want to focus on your hip and thigh area.

It is very important to remember that spot toning alone does not work. Spot toning is the term for exercise that concentrates merely on one area rather than focusing on the body as a whole. A good example of this is someone who does 200 sit ups every night and still moans that they have fat across their tummy. This is because their body shape is made up of both fat and muscle. Fat does not turn into muscle and muscle does not turn into fat. What does happen is that when you work muscle it

# of staying active

becomes firmer and stronger and when you work harder you use up calories which can help reduce your fat stores. So if you are to improve the appearance of your hips and thighs you need to adopt the following two-pronged approach:

- Firm your muscles
- Reduce your fat stores

These two missions, when they are put into practice together, will make the biggest impact on how you look. Whilst it is true that spot toning alone will not work, it does help, however, to take up a sport or activity that uses the lower body for a lot of its work. Such activities and sports include running, cycling, step classes, tennis, skipping, hill climbing, hiking and cross-country skiing.

ideas to try

Here are some exercise routines that you can try out yourself at home. Both activities tend to be aerobic in nature, i.e. they use oxygen to keep the body supplied with energy and, in this way, you will not only work the lower body muscles but burn body fat as well.

▼ 5-minute stair workout

If you can't get to a step class, try using your staircase at home instead.

Instructions

1 Walk up and down the stairs twice to warm up.

2 Run up the stairs and walk back down. Then run up the stairs, 2 at a time, and walk back down.

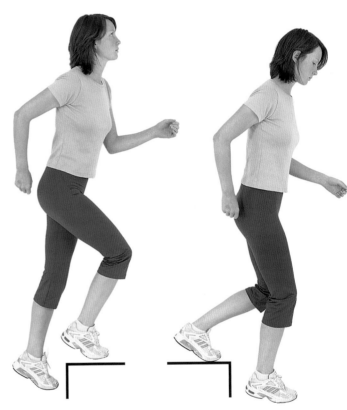

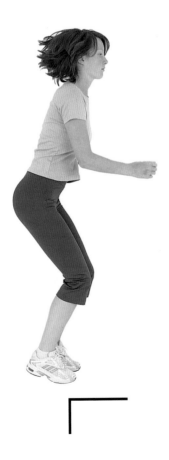

3 Jump with both feet onto the first step and step back down 5 times.

4 Now jump up 2 stairs (place your hand on the banisters for balance) and step back down 5 times.

5 Place your hands on the third stair and then jump your feet up and down on the first step 5 times.

6 Repeat the whole sequence and finish by gently walking up and down the first step to recover.

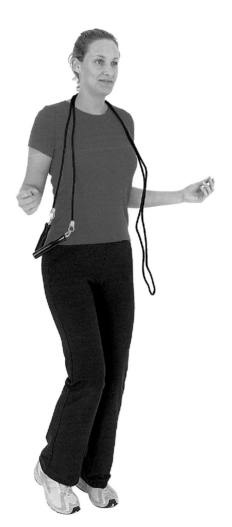

◀ 5-minute skipping routine
Instructions

1 Grab a skipping rope and hold it in one hand, walking and then jogging on the spot to warm up.

2 Now place the rope around your neck and skip with your feet as if you had the rope in your hands.

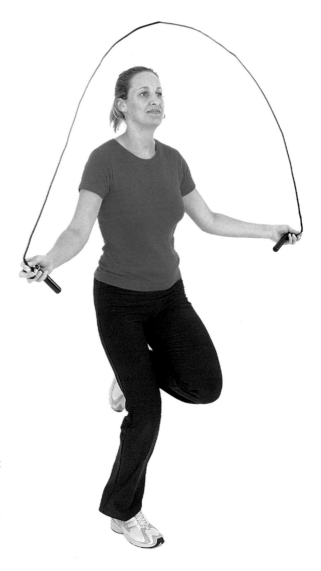

3 Hold the rope in both hands and try to skip with alternate feet. Lift your feet just off the floor and let the rope swing underneath. Try to keep the movement smooth. You should not jump too high but just skip from one foot to another.

4 Aim to do 1 minute's skipping without a break, then skip forwards and backwards. As you get more proficient at skipping, try turning around as you skip or even flick the rope twice over as you jump!

walking

One of the easiest ways to boost your circulation and tone your lower body is walking. This is an easy, low-impact way to gain all the different aspects of fitness including a shaping up of the lower body. Many people who have attempted longer walks of, say, 13.1 miles (half-marathon) or 26.2 miles (marathon) have reported a shaping up and weight loss from around their hips and legs.

We Can All Walk

Virtually all types of people can get something out of a walking programme. Even if you are older or have not done anything active for a while, a walking programme can help. Even people with high blood pressure or diabetes can walk, as can those recovering from surgery or other types of treatment. The great thing about walking is it can be done anywhere and can start off very easy and become gradually harder as your fitness and stamina improve.

The Benefits

Because walking is a social activity, you can include others and this will help to make it feel more like fun than a workout! Try to arrange to walk with someone if possible, preferably someone who can walk at around your pace and has similar (hip shaping) goals! As you begin to walk regularly you will notice that it can help relax and unwind you after a stressful day. It will not only tone your muscles but help you sleep better and give you feelings of well being as the endorphins get released. Overall you will feel brighter and fitter; fast walking can even help to control your appetite.

How to Get Started

The first thing to do is grab a friend and get out there! Anywhere is fine – roads and city streets or parks and fields. Warm up your feet and ankles before you start and then step out and chat as you go! Think of your walk initially in three parts:

- Do the first 5 minutes at a slow pace.
- Increase your speed for the next 5 minutes.
- Use the last 5 minutes to slow the pace down again as you cool down.

Try to walk at least twice a week – more if you can. Over the weeks, you can gradually increase the time (and therefore distance) that you walk so the walks will become progressively more challenging. If you progress things in this incremental way, perhaps adding 5 minutes on to each walk you do, then you will avoid any severe stiffness or muscle soreness as your body will have time to repair and adapt to the new demands.

Safety

Keeping safe is something to be aware of as you begin to walk further and faster. Be aware of the following guidelines:

- Make sure you have the appropriate footwear. Your shoes should be relatively new (not over a year old) and well cushioned with a bendable sole. Go to a technical running shop where they can check the fit for your shoes and suggest a shoe if you have a tendency to pronate.
- Wear bright reflective clothing if you are going to walk in the evenings. Buy some reflective strips to sew onto your favourite walking jackets and T-shirts. Always walk with someone, never alone.
- Don't wear jewellery or head phones when out walking and keep your mobile phone out of sight in your bum bag.
- Keep observant and take a note of any landmarks that you have passed just in case you get lost!

51

Weekly Walking Programme

	Warm up	Fast walk	Cool down	Total time
Week 1	Walk slowly 5 mins	Walk briskly 5 mins	Walk slowly 5 mins	15 mins
Week 2	Walk slowly 5 mins	Walk briskly 8 mins	Walk slowly 5 mins	18 mins
Week 3	Walk slowly 5 mins	Walk briskly 11 mins	Walk slowly 5 mins	21 mins
Week 4	Walk briskly 5 mins	Walk slowly 14 mins	Walk slowly 5 mins	24 mins
Week 5	Walk slowly 5 mins	Walk briskly 17 mins	Walk slowly 5 mins	27 mins
Week 6	Walk slowly 5 mins	Walk briskly 20 mins	Walk slowly 5 mins	30 mins
Week 7	Walk slowly 5 mins	Walk briskly 23 mins	Walk slowly 5 mins	33 mins
Week 8	Walk slowly 5 mins	Walk briskly 26 mins	Walk slowly 5 mins	36 mins
Week 9+	Walk slowly 5 mins	Walk briskly 30 mins	Walk slowly 5 mins	40 mins

▶ Ankle Warm Up

Before you start your slow 5-minute walk, warm up your ankles.

Instructions

1 March on the spot briefly, pushing your toes down first and then rolling through the foot onto the heel.

2 Tap toe-heel, toe-heel on one foot 10 times, then do the same with the other foot.

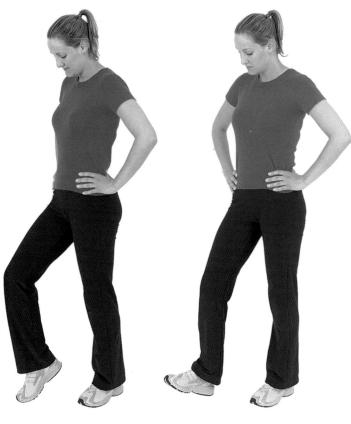

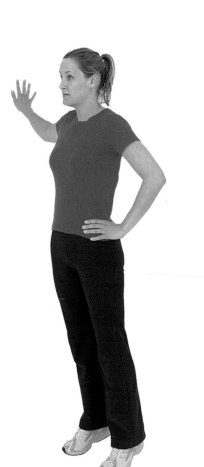

3 Hold onto a wall and raise yourself up onto both toes (as high as you can) and then lower your heels to the floor. Perform 8 raises and lowers, then shake out your calves and repeat.

4 Take one leg out behind you (as if you are in a lunge position) and press the heel into the floor. Now push the back heel off the floor and press it back down again. Repeat on each leg 8 times.

Walking Technique

When walking, your shoulders should be slightly back with your arms moving with your legs. Swing your arms forwards and back as you walk. Don't keep them still or straight, just hanging down by your sides. This will slow you down and you may find your hands swelling as you walk. Instead, bend your arms and swing them to add speed and balance to your walk. Nor should you allow your bent arms to swing from side to side – only forwards and back.

Keep your head up so that you can look around at your surroundings and see what is coming up ahead. This is good posture which will help you to breathe properly and prevent an aching neck or shoulders.

Try not to lean too far forwards or too far back. This can result in back or hip pain so try to stand up straight (unless you're battling against a very strong wind!) and keep your shoulders relaxed. Think about walking tall: lift your torso out of your ribcage and keep your abdominal muscles tight.

With your feet you should be hitting the heel of the foot to the floor first and rolling through the foot onto the metatarsals and then pushing off behind you with the toes. You should not hear a slapping noise as you walk – if this is the case, your shoes may be too inflexible or you may need to make a conscious effort to roll through the feet. Keep your feet pointing forwards and don't step too wide.

Some people have a tendency to over stride, reaching out with their front foot as they try to speed up their pace. This doesn't really help speed and can lead to an odd gait hurting shins or feet. The power in walking comes from pushing off with your back foot, so when you want to speed up, take shorter, faster steps and really roll through your foot and give a good push off with the toe. This will give you greater speed and a longer stride at the back.

What to Wear

Make sure you wear clothes that are practical when walking. Start with a hat. It will keep your body heat in so that you warm up faster (leading to better overall performance) and will protect you from the sun and rain.

Wear comfortable, multiple layers so that you can strip off a layer as you become warm and put it back on if you cool down. The layer next to your skin should be a proper exercise fabric such as Coolmax or polypropylene which will filter away sweat from your body, rather than cotton which will hold it next to the skin. The next layer should be insulating, such as a jumper or sweatshirt, to keep in the warmth. The top layer should be a waterproof, windproof jacket which is easily removable

A bum bag is probably the best way to carry your water bottle and snack provisions (if you are doing a long session). It will sit comfortably at the small of your back as you walk. Some people drink more than others on long walks, and the recommended sip rate is: drink a cup of water every 20–30 minutes and drink 2 cups of water when you finish.

interval training
workout

Some people just don't have the time to put in hours of walking, so if you are looking for a faster, tougher solution then try the 16-minute principle for interval training. This is a short, sharp, intense cardiovascular routine which works you hard and fast but gets great results. It has one simple principle which helps to focus you and ensures you always work your hardest. This technique has evolved from body builders who want to do only the minimum cardiovascular training, partly because they wish to spend all their time building muscle mass and partly because they believe a too long CV session will eat into their muscle stores. Normal exercisers don't need to worry about such technicalities but you can learn from their commitment to hard, fast workouts to ensure that you burn calories and really challenge the muscles.

Exercise Bike Workout

Find a workout you can do and repeat time and time again. The easiest kind of training is on a workout bike.

1 Set the resistance on the bike to a low level. Next set your stop watch to beep after 16 minutes.

2 Now start pedalling! Your aim in the first session is to go at a pace that you can comfortably do, and keep up, for 16 minutes.

3 At the end of this time, check and note down the distance you covered. Your task the next time you repeat this workout is simply to cover a greater distance than you did last time. That's all there is to it! Your second workout will be exactly the same resistance and exactly the same length of time as before – 16 minutes. However, the distance you cover will increase as you work progressively harder.

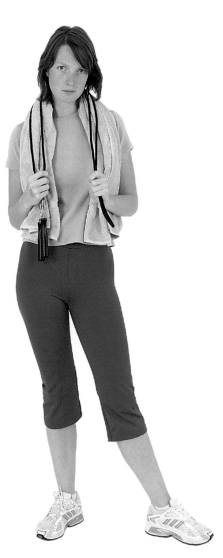

Other Workouts

If you don't have an exercise bike, don't worry.
You simply need to find a workout method that
provides a means of recording your efforts. You
could use skipping, running, walking, stepping or
a rowing machine or skier. All these workouts will
allow you to push your limits and achieve more
within the same time frame. Your best choice for
a workout would be an exercise that uses the
legs heavily as this will benefit the hips and
thighs. Here are some ideas for you to try out:

- Time 16 minutes on a rowing machine. Next
time do more strokes or a greater distance in
the same time.
- Set off walking or running and note the
distance you cover in 16 minutes. Next time
walk or run further in the same time.
- If you skip, note how many skips you do in
16 minutes. Put in different moves and note
how many of each move, e.g. double skips,
you fit in. Next time beat that score!
- If you are using a step, keep a note of how
many step ups (of different sorts) you manage
in 16 minutes. Next time, beat that score!

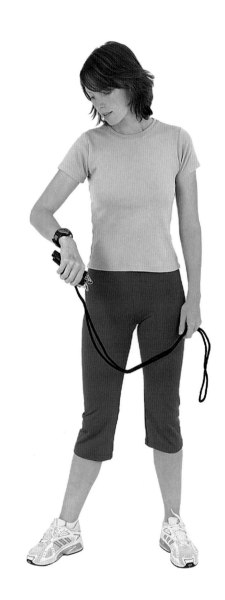

55

This is a short, sharp, intense
cardiovascular routine which
works you hard and fast but
gets great results.

part 4

start your workout

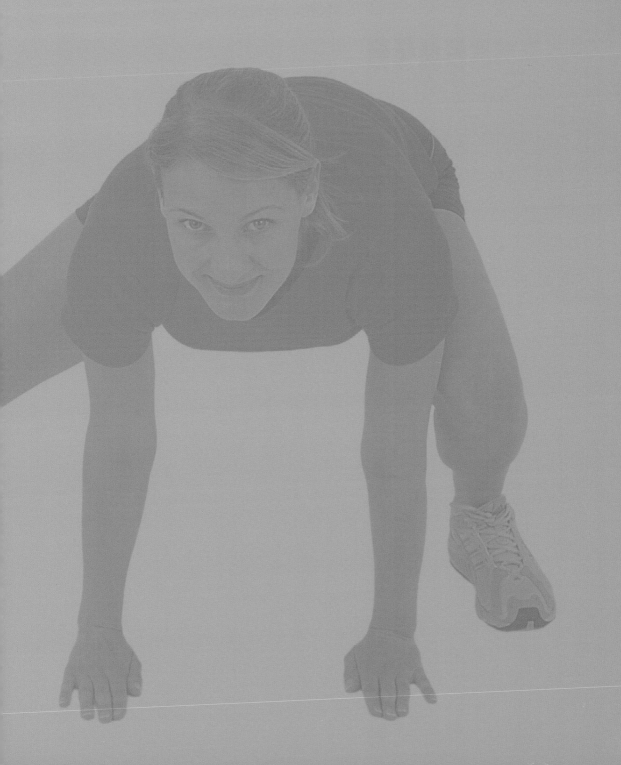

make the most of the

In this book you have a versatile and varied programme of 10-minute workouts, which, if performed regularly, will really tone up and shape your hips and thighs – as well as making you feel fitter all over!

You should make an effort to put aside some time on a regular basis for your hip and thigh workouts. Unless you allocate some formal time for your exercise plan, the chances are it won't happen. So sit down with a pen and paper or your diary before you start your routine and really map out when you can fit in 10 or 20 minutes for hip and thigh exercises every few days.

programme

59

Think of some convenient times during the day when you can fit in a few informal exercises on a regular basis. What about when you get up in the morning? A few repetitions of an exercise might get the blood flowing and wake you up. Or what about just before you go to bed? Doing a couple of exercises and a stretch might help you to sleep better. Alternatively, what about just before you take a bath or a shower? If you are committed, there are probably several opportunities in the day when you can do some toning and improve the appearance of your hips and thighs.

before you start

Make sure that you are prepared mentally and physically to begin each workout session – then you will get the best results. If you have not done any formal exercise for over six months you should check with your doctor before starting a home programme without supervision.

Safety Tips

Before you start your workout, read through the following safety guidelines.

- Make sure you have plenty of space available for your workout. It should be free of clutter and well ventilated.
- Place a towel by your side in readiness for some of the exercises and turn on a music system playing your favourite tune.
- Always keep a glass of water handy so that you can sip in between exercises. In this way, you will keep yourself hydrated as you work out.
- If you are cold at the beginning of your workout, wear a sweat shirt when you start your warm up to help heat up the muscles. Make sure you are wearing layers that you can strip off as you begin to warm up.
- You should always be very warm before attempting the stretching part of this programme. Muscles will not benefit from stretching unless they are warm and pliable so always make sure that the hip and thigh stretching programmes follow either the toning sections or the CV sections, such as the rebounder workout (see page 75).
- After working out, be sure to drink regularly throughout the day (you should have 8–10 good-sized glasses of water), and eat within two hours of working out to prevent blood sugar levels dropping.

Wear layers of clothing when you train. You should start off really warm, then strip back the layers as you begin to sweat.

Sample Programmes

These programmes can be done in any combination so long as you don't do the stretching when you are cold, so mix and match the various elements of the book to the time you have available. Below are some sample weeks you might like to try. In each case, Sunday is a rest day. As you progress from week 1 to week 6, gradually increase the time and intensity of the workouts.

Suggested Weekly Workouts

61

Week 1: Easy

Monday	Tuesday	Wednesday	Thursday	Friday	Saturday
Warm up	Warm up	Warm up	Warm up	Warm up	Warm up
Walking	Rebounder	Walking	Rebounder	Walking	Hip stretches
Hip toners	Thigh toners	Massage	Yoga	Thigh stretches	Cool down
Cool down	Cool down	Cool down	Cool down	Cool down	

Now gradually increase the time and intensity of the workouts throughout weeks 2 to 5.

Week 6: Hard

Monday	Tuesday	Wednesday	Thursday	Friday	Saturday
Skin brushing	Skin brushing	Skin brushing	Skin brushing	Skin brushing	Skin brushing
Warm up	Warm up	Warm up	Warm up	Warm up	Warm up
Walking	Interval training	Rebounder	Walking	Rebounder	Walking
Hip toners	Thigh toners	Massage	Yoga	Thigh toners	Hip toners
Hip stretches	Thigh stretches	Hip stretches	Thigh toners	Cool down	Cool down
Cool down	Cool down	Cool down	Cool down		

prepare your body

Warming up before you perform your major hip and thigh exercises is very important. Even when you do only 10 minutes of thigh exercises, you still need to ready the body for exercise. Warming up is exactly what it says – moving around with the objective of creating an internal heat which enables the body to work more efficiently.

As you begin to march, for example, and you pick up your knees and pump your arms, you are using numerous muscles and working a variety of joints. As the joints work, the synovial fluid between the surfaces is warmed and liquefies to allow the bones to move more smoothly against each other. As you move your whole body, each joint and muscle is warmed, thereby allowing a greater range of movement which, in turn, prepares the body for further movement. As you continue to move your body, you can also practise some of the more precise movements you may be doing in the bulk of your workout. Proper warming up helps prevent cramps which can occur if you are concentrating too much on a particular move.

The exercises that follow focus on the lower body, including the joints of the hip and knee, so you need all the benefits of a proper warm up. Even though you will be targeting only the lower body, the whole body needs to be warm before starting the exercises.

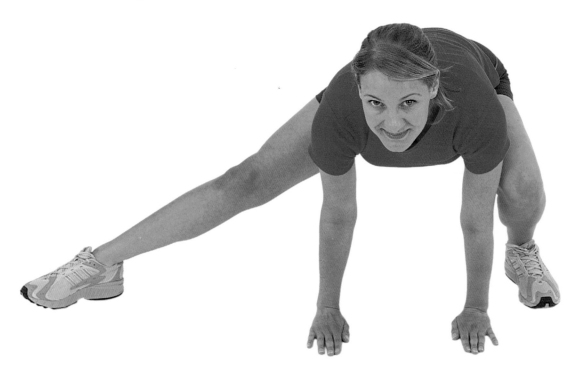

Even if you do only 10 minutes of thigh exercises, you still need to ready the body for exercise.

Benefits of a Good Warm Up

The beneficial effects of performing a proper warm up include the following:

- Increased body temperature means that all the systems of the body are prepared. As core temperature increases, the blood vessels dilate, thus allowing a good flow of blood and reducing the work for the heart.
- When muscle temperature is increased, the muscles become more pliant and can contract forcefully and relax readily. This guards against pulls and muscle strains. It also means that the muscles will be at their optimum for working intensely, to gain strength and stamina.
- Increased blood temperature is thought to allow a greater release of oxygen into the working muscles.
- As you warm up the body, hormonal changes occur which allow more carbohydrates and fatty acids to be available for energy production.
- The readying of the body occurs mentally, too. As you begin your warm up you can start to focus on the work you will be doing. You can practise concentration and leave all problems of the day behind you as you focus purely on the task in hand. Not only will this mean that your workout is concentrated and thoughtful but you will also end your session feeling mentally refreshed after having thought of nothing else for 15 minutes!

Which Exercises?

Warm up exercises can include any movements that are relatively simple and use the large muscles of the body. With some sports or workouts, a warm up may just be a simpler or slower form of some of the main activities before increasing the intensity. Stretching exercises are not warm up exercises so don't put these at the beginning of any of your programmes. A muscle – indeed, the whole body – needs to warm before you start to stretch out. A warm up should include exercises that mobilize the joints of the body and get the whole frame working.

63

warm up

H ere are some suggested warm up exercises but you can add your own simple dance steps and linking movements as well, if wished. Put on some music, if it helps, when you're performing these moves and enjoy yourself as you get warm!

▶ **Pump it up**

Instructions

1 Start with both feet on the ground and your hands by your sides.

2 Lift one heel and then the other as you alternate your feet, pressing each heel as high as you can to warm up your feet and ankles.

3 Now pump your arms to get the heat going in your upper body, too.

4 As you pick up the speed of this movement, you can swing the hips slightly from side to side – have fun with this!

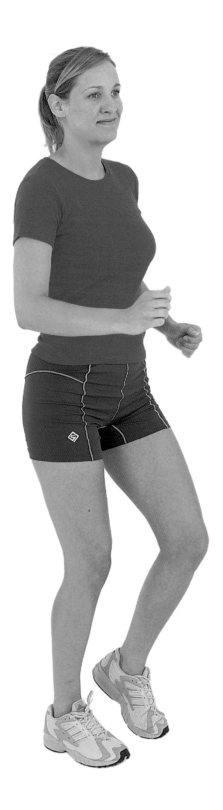

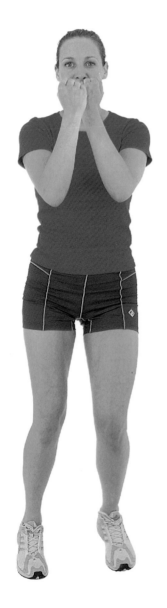

◄ Boxer's skips
Instructions

1 Rise up onto the balls of your feet and start to bounce from one foot to the other. Hold your hands up by your mouth (because that's what boxers do to protect themselves) and stay on your toes to help you bounce.

2 Skip from side to side.

3 Keep jigging for 2–3 minutes and you will really feel the heat!

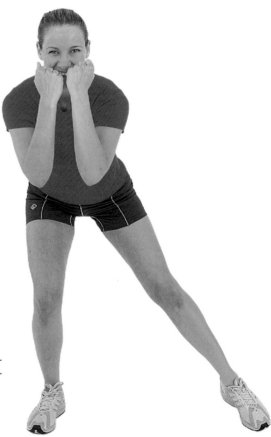

Imagine you are ducking an opponent who is throwing a punch at you!

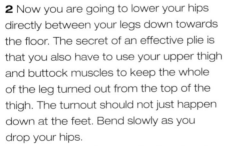

◀ Plies

Plies, or low bending movements, are one of the fastest ways of warming up the legs and lower body.

Instructions

1 For this plie stand with your legs wide apart and your feet slightly turned out.

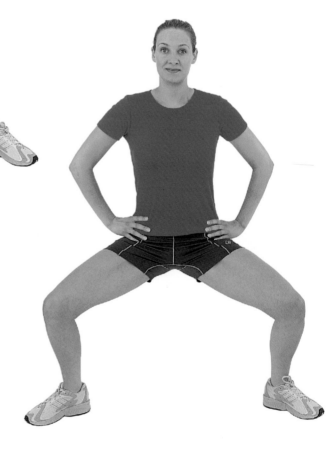

2 Now you are going to lower your hips directly between your legs down towards the floor. The secret of an effective plie is that you also have to use your upper thigh and buttock muscles to keep the whole of the leg turned out from the top of the thigh. The turnout should not just happen down at the feet. Bend slowly as you drop your hips.
3 Now squeeze the muscles to return to standing.
4 Perform this move 15 times, then shake your legs out!

▾ Growing tree

Warm those legs up even more as you do a 3-step deep bend in this move.

Instructions

1 Stand with your feet hip width apart.
2 Now bend your knees and touch the floor.
3 Next touch your knees.
4 Reach up towards the ceiling, as high as you can. You should be on your tiptoes with your stomach pulled in and up, reaching and stretching as high as you can.
5 Bend your knees and go back down to touch the floor.
6 Repeat this move 8–10 times, then take a breather while marching on the spot.
7 Repeat the 10 repetitions again to really build up some heat!

67

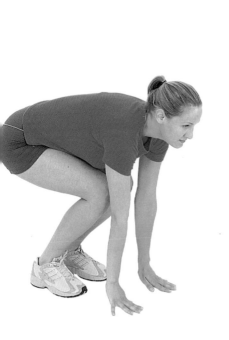
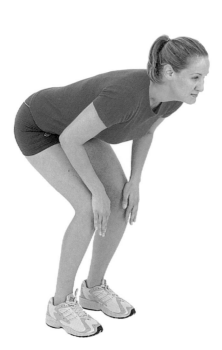
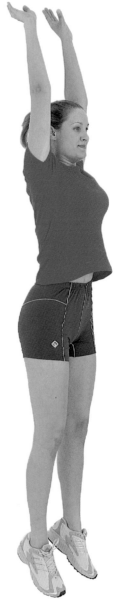

▸ Torso toner
Instructions

1 Warm up the middle of the body as this will generate heat throughout! Stand with your hands on your hips and move the hips in one direction and then the other.

2 Push the hips, with your hands, round in a big circle one way and then the other.

3 Bend your knees for one circle, then straighten them for the other. Have fun!

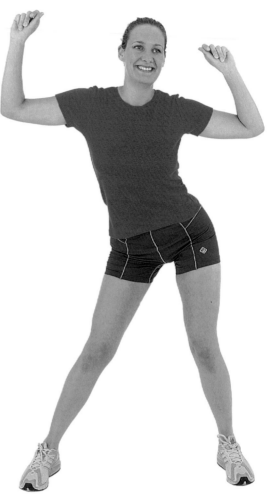

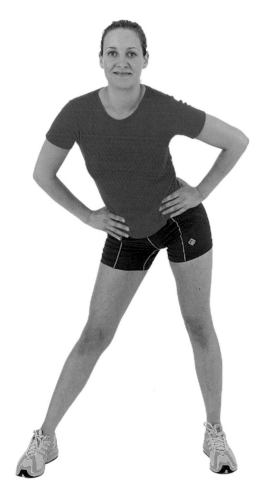

Vary the speeds: try doing it really slowly, then really fast.

▼ Half jacks

Really up the heat now by performing some half jacks. These will mobilize your hips and legs.

Instructions

1 Stand on both feet and then push off one leg and squat to one side. Take the squat as low as feels comfortable.

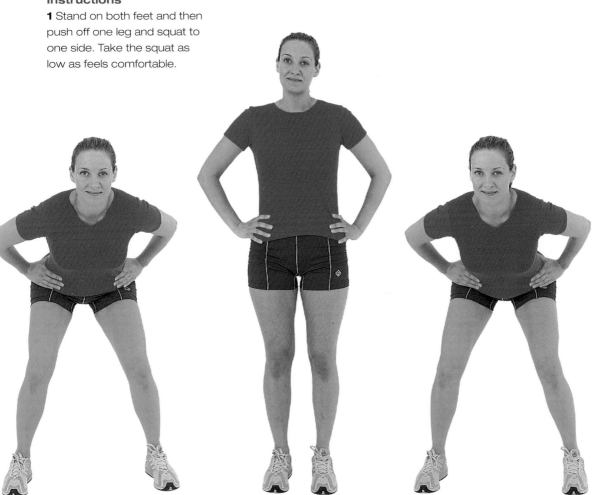

2 Now push off with the other foot and squat to the other side.
3 Alternate sides with a skip in between for 10–12 squats.

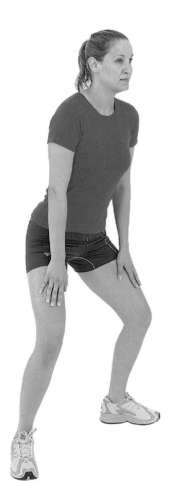

◀ Back plies

These moves will mobilize the spine and upper half of the body.

Instructions

1 Repeat the plie you did earlier but hold the downward position.

2 Now place your hands on your knees and press one shoulder forward (with a straight arm) and pull the other shoulder back behind. Hollow it by dropping your head and stretching out your back.

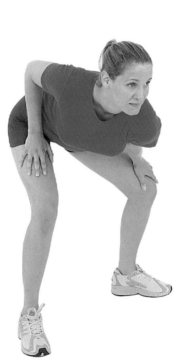

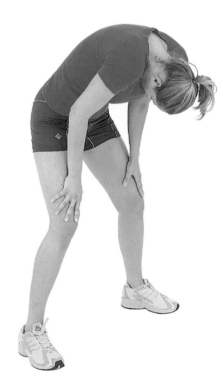

3 Press one shoulder forward, then the other, using a smooth motion.

4 Press the back straight and then hollow it by dropping your head and stretching out your back.

▼ Leg swings

Instructions

1 Mobilize the hip joints by standing on one leg. Place your hand on the wall for balance.

2 Now swing your outside leg forwards and then backwards. Do 20 swings.

3 Change legs and repeat on the other side.

71

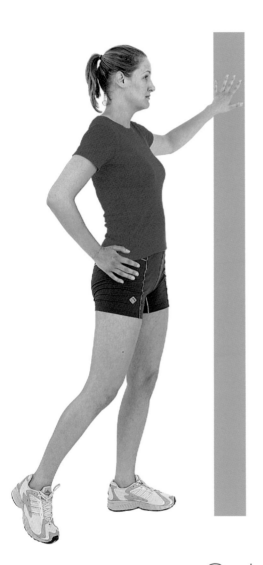
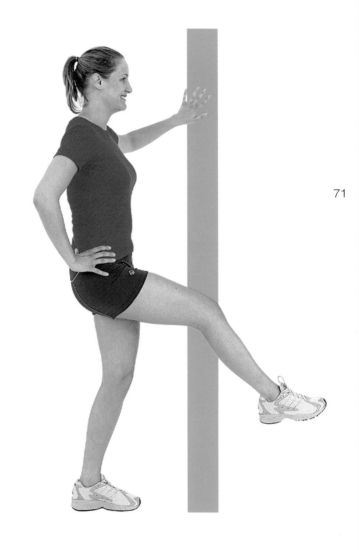

Swing your leg low and loosely in the hip, just to warm the joint.

Rebounding

A good cardiovascular system will keep the skin and muscle around the hips and thighs looking smooth. Rebounding exercises will boost your circulation and fitness. You need a mini trampoline or trampette (usually called a rebounder), which uses gravitational pull to assist your movement. By aiding the upward motion of the body and cushioning its descent, it provides the perfect G-force for training safely. This use of gravity stimulates body cells and boosts circulation without putting any stress on the body. Trampettes also offer good shock absorption properties and thus can be very useful for people with joint problems. In addition, balancing on a trampette uses the hip and thigh muscles quite intensely.

rebounder exercises

T he following exercises can be done on the floor if you cannot get hold of a rebounder. The impact of some exercises will be greater if you do them on the floor so try to find a wooden floor that has a little give in it. You could even try using your bed – but check its strength first!

▶ Pulsing

One of the first moves to learn when you first climb onto your rebounder is the pulser or 'health bounce'.

Instructions

1 Stand with both feet flat on the mat and then start to lift first one heel and then the other (see warm up, page 64). Work your arms back and forwards too and you will soon get into a rhythm as the mat bends with your weight. Keep this going for a few minutes as you breathe in through your nose and out through your mouth.

2 Now press both heels flat to the mat and start to bounce with both feet. Allow a slight articulation in your feet as you bounce; don't be tempted to lift the heels.
3 Keep bouncing for 5 minutes. Continue to breathe in through your nose and out through your mouth.

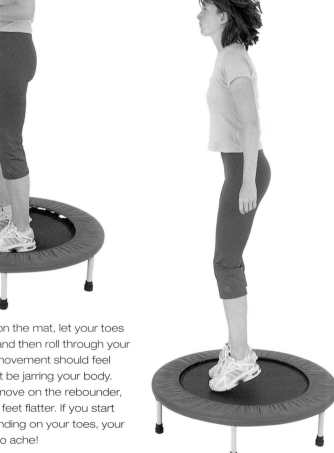

4 If you are doing this on the mat, let your toes touch the ground first and then roll through your feet to the heels. The movement should feel soft and you should not be jarring your body.
5 If you are doing the move on the rebounder, you need to keep your feet flatter. If you start lifting your heels and landing on your toes, your calves will really begin to ache!

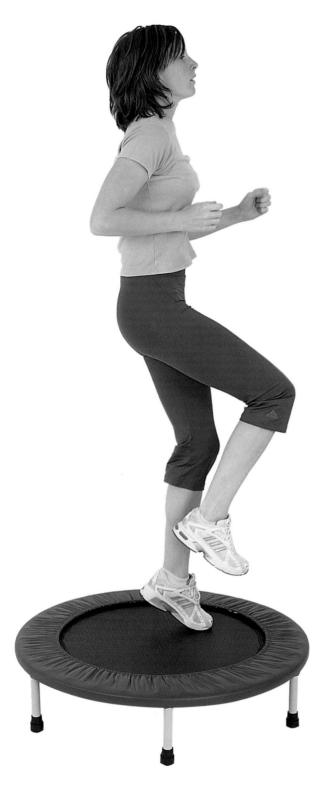

◀ Energetic jog

The great thing about the rebounder is that it makes jogging really easy. It absorbs the impact of the running yet gets the blood flowing fast at the same time.

Instructions

1 Step onto the rebounder and stand with both feet hip width apart.

2 Now start off by lifting first one heel and then the other and swinging your arms. This will help accustom you to the moving surface on the trampette. Keep doing this for several minutes.

3 Push your hips out to the sides and make the movement bigger as you become more at ease with the motion.

4 Now start to pick up your feet and lift your heels behind you as you move into a jog. Keep breathing and try to keep jogging, becoming faster and more energetic as you go!

5 This move will warm up the whole body and really get the blood flowing. Keep it going for 10–12 minutes.

▼ Tuck jumps

Instructions

1 Bounce in the centre of the rebounder once again.

2 This time you are going to take off with both feet and spring upwards. Use your arms to help the upward movement and, as you lift off the mat, try to tuck your knees up in front of you. Keep your head lifted as you try to lift your knees and pull in on the abdominals to help lift your legs.

3 Land and repeat the jump immediately.

4 If you are doing this move on the floor rather than the rebounder, you may need a break after 4 consecutive jumps!

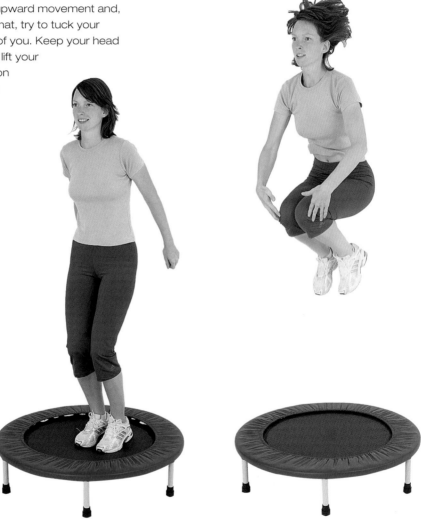

Build a routine

Try alternating the tuck jumps and star jumps with the jogging and health bounce moves you have learned. In this way, you will develop a 10–15 minute routine you can use every other day to boost the blood flow and wake up that circulation each morning!

Getting higher

Now you can begin to experiment a little more actively with your rebounder. Try these moves to really get your circulation – and adrenalin – going! You can perform the moves on the floor also, but be sure to land going through the foot and bending the knees softly to avoid any jarring of the body.

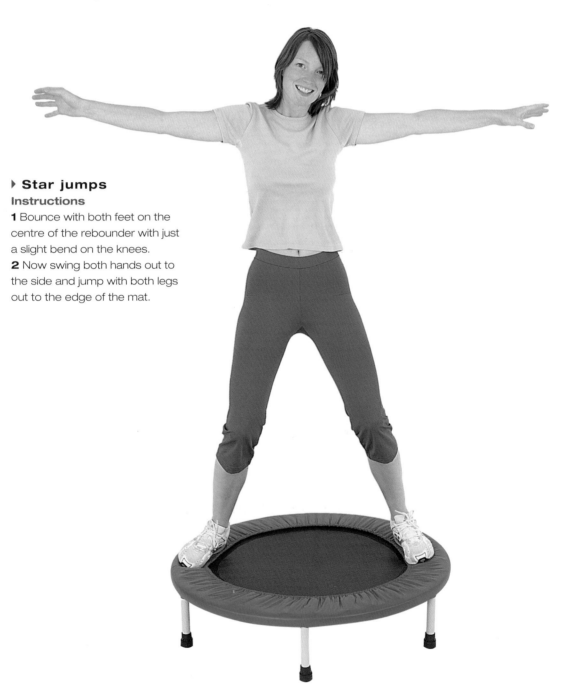

▶ Star jumps

Instructions

1 Bounce with both feet on the centre of the rebounder with just a slight bend on the knees.

2 Now swing both hands out to the side and jump with both legs out to the edge of the mat.

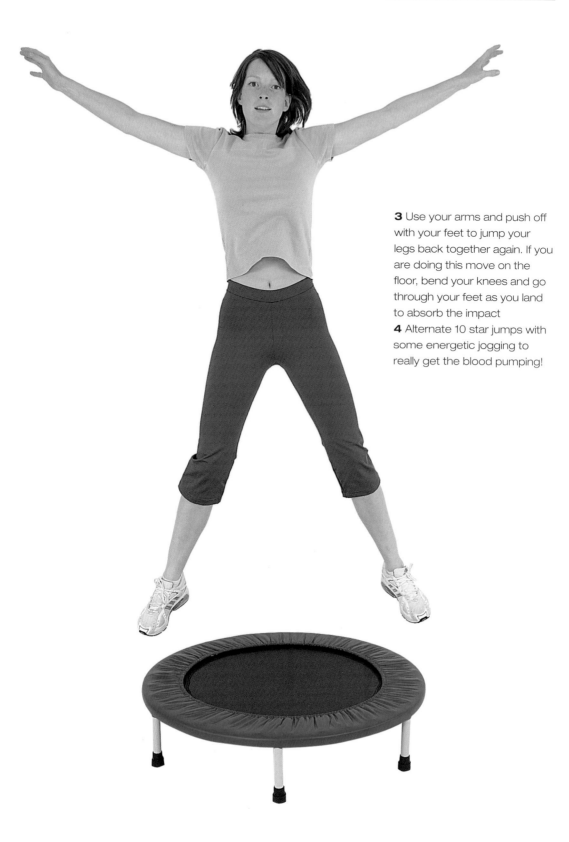

3 Use your arms and push off with your feet to jump your legs back together again. If you are doing this move on the floor, bend your knees and go through your feet as you land to absorb the impact

4 Alternate 10 star jumps with some energetic jogging to really get the blood pumping!

yoga booster

Devotees claim yoga helps boost circulation and reduce stress levels. Stress can restrict blood flow, as can a sluggish system, so perform some basic yoga moves to boost a slow metabolism which collects fat around your hips and thighs. These involve twisting and bending which, it is claimed, massage muscles and internal organs. Working hard in the sustained poses of the Ashtanga postures will help to flush oxygen-rich blood to the working muscles and encourage cell repair and growth. One of the key tenets of yoga is synchronizing your breath with each movement, helping to oxygenate the blood and reducing stress on body systems. You need to perform yoga daily to improve the strength and appearance of the lower body.

How to use this sequence

The aim of the following series of moves, known in their totality as the Sun Salutation A, is to build a serious heat within the body. Try to learn the sequence slowly, step by step, adding a new move each time you have got to grips with the last. There is a lot to think about in each move, so take your time and build up the sequence over a week or so. When you are in each position, try to concentrate and focus on all the different aspects of the move that you need to correct. You should check constantly that all the different parts of your body are in the right places. This will focus your mind and work the body harder.

Sun salutation A

Try to learn, by heart, the following sequence which is the basic 'warm up' of yoga. A powerful and tiring routine, it will leave you feeling revived although you have worked your lower body hard.

▶ Position 1

Instructions

1 Stand with your feet together, arms by your sides, and gaze straight ahead.
2 Inhale deeply and slowly.
3 Raise your arms out to the sides and over your head to touch both palms together. Look up at your finger tips. Your thighs should be pulled up.
4 Reach up as high as you can, feeling as though you are pulling throughout the entire length of your body.

81

▶ Position 2
Instructions

1 Exhale slowly.

2 Lean forwards and lower the palms of your hands to the floor. As you lean, keep your legs straight and thighs pulled up.

3 When your palms are on the floor, tuck your head into your knees.

4 If you cannot achieve this move, don't worry, simply bend your knees as you lean over and keep them bent as you tuck your head in.

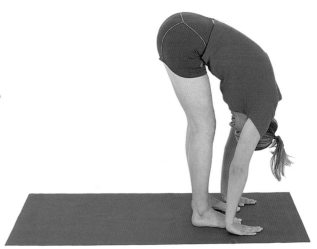

▶ Position 3
Instructions

1 Inhale deeply.

2 Look upward but keep your hands flat on the floor. Straighten your legs, if you can – if not, keep them bent – and try to lengthen your back and neck.

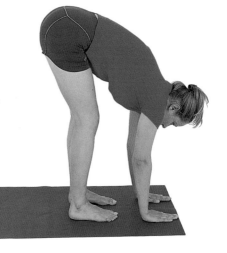

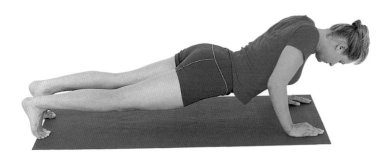

◀ Position 4
Instructions

1 Exhale deeply.

2 Walk your legs back until you are in a push up position.

3 Bend your arms to lower your body until it is just off the floor. If you don't have the strength to lower from that position, bend your knees and lower your body to the floor from there.

▶ Position 5

Instructions

1 Inhale deeply.

2 Roll over the tops of your feet and press your hips forwards, lifting your body onto your hands and resting on the tops of your feet. Ideally, your knees and hips should not touch the ground.

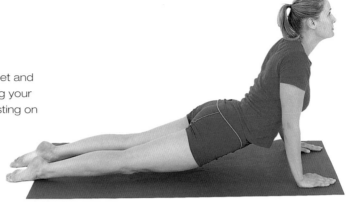

3 This position can be very difficult for beginners or people with tight ankles or backs. If so, adopt an easier position by keeping your knees on the floor and arching back as much as you can.

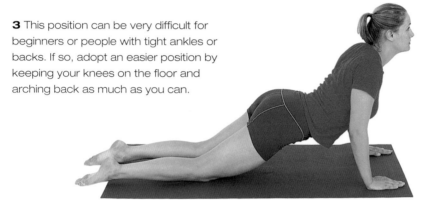

83

▼ Position 6

Instructions

1 Exhale deeply, then take 5 breaths. Push up, leading with your bottom and pressing on your arms to form an upside-down 'V' shape (the downward facing dog position). Stay like this for 5 whole breaths, breathing in deeply through your nose and out through the mouth.

2 Press your hips up into the air as you press your chest down towards the floor. Press your armpits, too, towards the floor so that you feel the stretch in your shoulders as you straighten and lengthen your upper back

3 Try to press your heel to the floor – you may not be able to do this due to the tension felt in the hamstrings at the back of your legs. Your feet should be parallel and about as far apart as your hip bones.

4 In this position, you are constantly working, pressing one end of the body away from the other. You should also be pulling up on the abdominal muscles and the inner pelvic floor muscles. All this work should really build up a heat inside you and will really boost blood flow as your body demands oxygen.

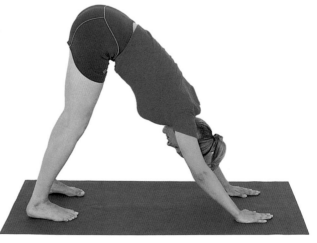

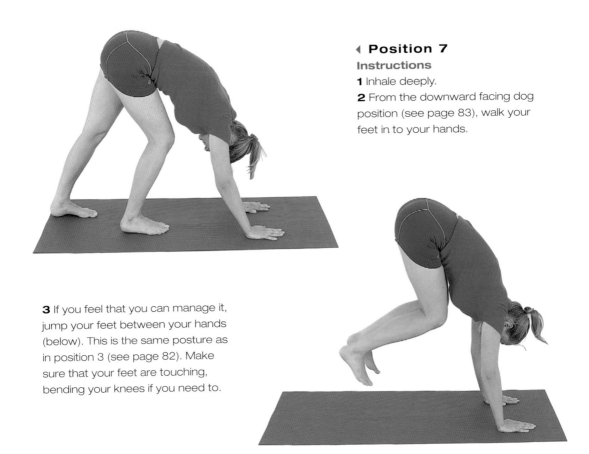

◀ **Position 7**

Instructions

1 Inhale deeply.

2 From the downward facing dog position (see page 83), walk your feet in to your hands.

3 If you feel that you can manage it, jump your feet between your hands (below). This is the same posture as in position 3 (see page 82). Make sure that your feet are touching, bending your knees if you need to.

▶ **Position 8**

Instructions

1 Exhale deeply.

2 Once again, tuck your head in as far towards your knees as possible. Try to look at your navel. Bend your knees if you need to – as in position 2 (see page 82).

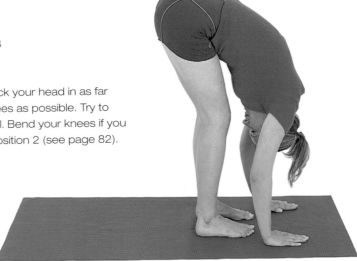

▶ Position 9

Instructions

1 Inhale deeply.

2 Reach all the way back up, leading with your arms and back, until you are standing.

3 Stretch your arms upwards above your head and lift up as high as you can through your body. Feel as though you are being pulled from your middle fingers up towards the sky. Your knee caps should be lifted, the pelvic floor pulled up and shoulders relaxed.

4 Lower your arms slowly and take 5 breaths to recover.

Summary

Once you have learned the moves, you can concentrate on making sure that you are breathing at the right moments as this will fill out the movement and aid hard work. Perform this whole sequence whenever you have a spare five minutes. Work through the sequence slowly and keep repeating it – up to 20 times! Each time you do it, you will notice that you get further and extend your flexibility and range of movement. When you have completed 20 sequences, you will be sweating profusely.

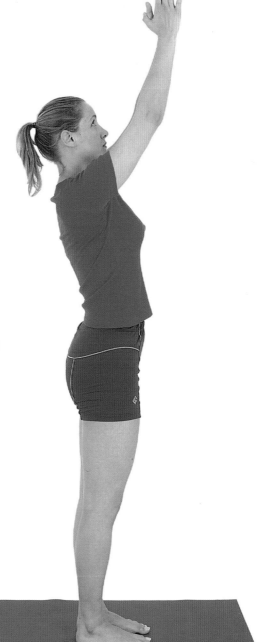

part 6

hip
exercises

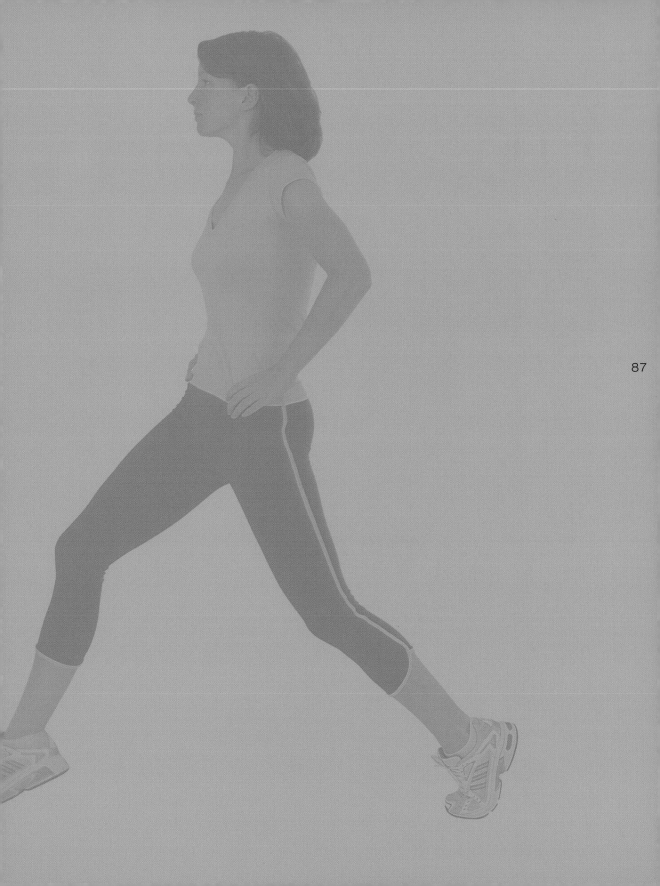

hip toners

Different muscles make up the hip area and give it its shape. Toning the buttocks at the back will improve the overall look of your hips. Try these toners to boost your bottom line. When you step and push behind you with force you are using the large buttock muscle: the gluteus maximus.

▶ **High-step hops**

Instructions

1 Use a high step or, if you don't have one handy, your stairs. Facing the step, step upwards onto the platform. (If you are using the stairs, step up two stairs.) As you step, use the body's force to propel you upwards into a jump.

2 Land back on the step and then place the other foot back on the floor.

3 Do 8 push offs on each foot, bending the knee of the push off leg to propel yourself off the ground.

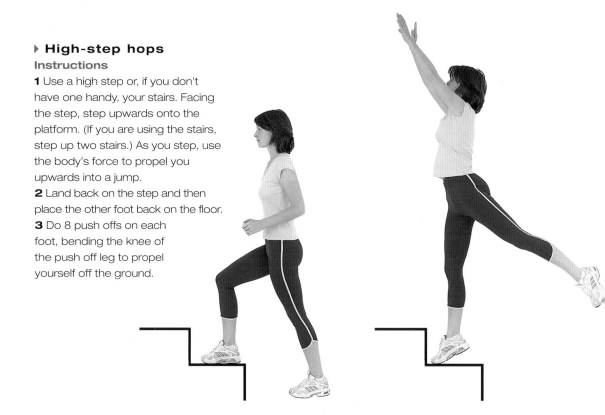

▶ High-step hop & kicks

Instructions

1 Use a high step or some stairs to do this move. Step onto the step and propel yourself into the air as before.
2 When you land, try to maintain your balance and don't replace your other foot.

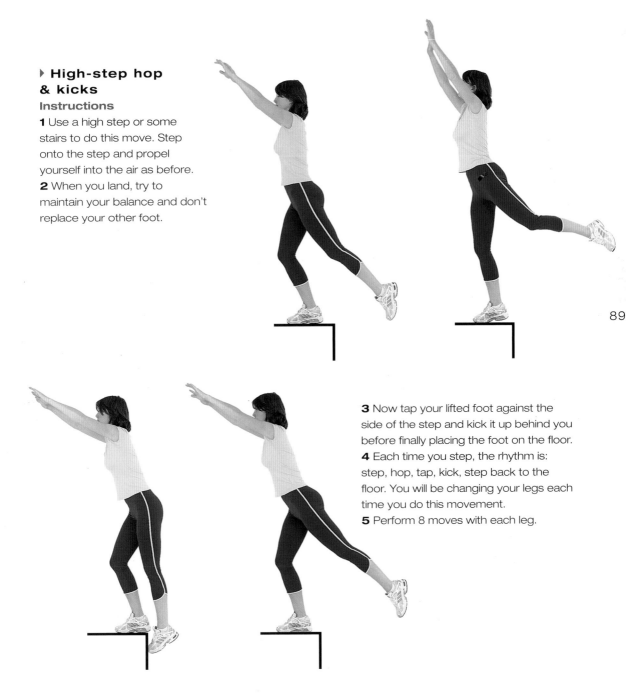

89

3 Now tap your lifted foot against the side of the step and kick it up behind you before finally placing the foot on the floor.
4 Each time you step, the rhythm is: step, hop, tap, kick, step back to the floor. You will be changing your legs each time you do this movement.
5 Perform 8 moves with each leg.

Work that buttock muscle by using the powerful drive of the back leg.

gluteus medius and minimus muscles

When you are running downhill, the gluteus minimus and medius muscles are under stress as they work to restrain the upper body from folding inwards. Use the following moves to work the gluteus medius and minimus.

▼ Lunge steps
Instructions

1 Stand with your feet together and step forwards, bending your front knee and lowering the groin towards the floor.
2 Push off with the back foot to swing this leg forwards to step into the lunge on the other side. Keep your hands on your hips.

3 Use this move to work your way across the room and then back again, keeping your upper body straight as you step and bend. Ensure that your toes don't go past your knee as you bend.

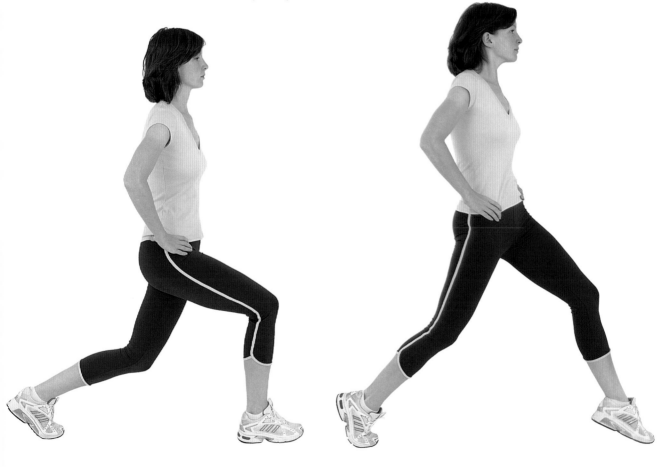

◀ Lunge steps with variations

Use the lunge step exercise but add some extra toning manoeuvres!

Instructions

1 Step and lunge, then push off with both feet equally so that you jump into the air.
2 Land and step with your other foot into your next lunge step.

3 Lower yourself even further and lean slightly forwards so that you can touch the floor with both hands – you will feel the work in the buttock of the front leg.
4 Come back to upright with your upper body, then repeat the whole sequence.

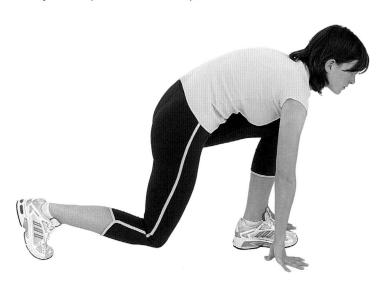

▼ Side pull backs

Instructions

1 Lie on one side, with your head resting on your arm and legs straight. Place the other hand on the floor in front of you to balance so you are lying on your side.

2 Now raise the leg on top, as high as you can. Hold it there for a second and then release it down again.

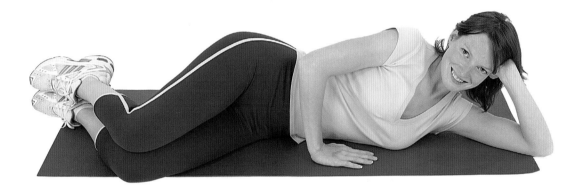

3 Try to keep the rest of the body still as you lift and lower the leg. You will feel this move in the side of your leg as well as around the hip.

4 Do 10 repetitions on one leg and then change sides and repeat with the other leg. Keep breathing regularly throughout the exercise.

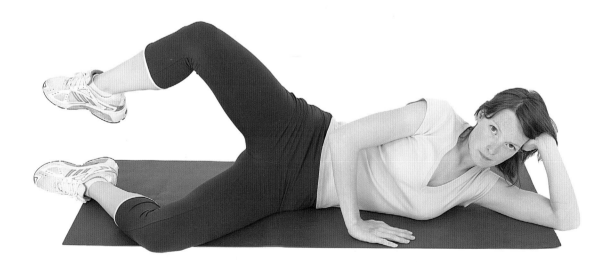

▼ Side curls (with partner)

Find a friend to help you with this exercise.
If no one is available, you can fix your feet
under a sofa to attempt the move.

Instructions

1 Lie on your side with the arm nearest
the floor wrapped across your body.
Have your partner straddle and
sit on your legs to stabilize
your position.

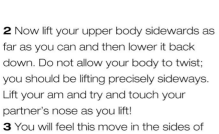

2 Now lift your upper body sidewards as
far as you can and then lower it back
down. Do not allow your body to twist;
you should be lifting precisely sideways.
Lift your am and try and touch your
partner's nose as you lift!
3 You will feel this move in the sides of
your stomach as well as in the hip area.
4 Try to do 10 repetitions and then repeat
on the other side.

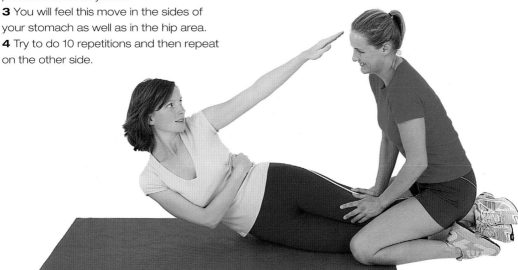

buttock muscles

The buttock muscles, particularly the large gluteus maximus, can work with greatest force if the body is bent forwards at the hip. The best exercises are those in which you extend your legs and hips at the same time.

▼ Length jumps
Instructions
1 Stand with your feet hip width apart.
2 Bend your knees and take your arms behind you almost to the ground. Your bottom is pushed out behind you and your back should be in a straight line from your hips to your head.

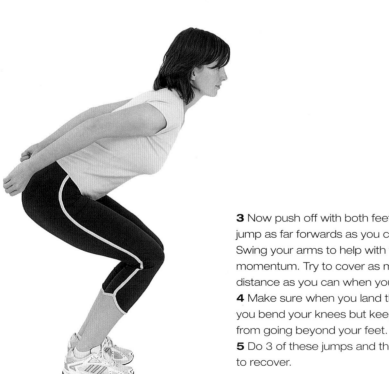

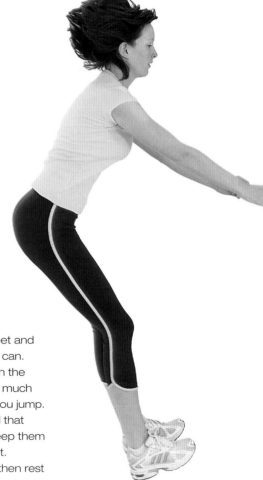

3 Now push off with both feet and jump as far forwards as you can. Swing your arms to help with the momentum. Try to cover as much distance as you can when you jump.
4 Make sure when you land that you bend your knees but keep them from going beyond your feet.
5 Do 3 of these jumps and then rest to recover.

‣ Squat jumps

Instructions

1 Stand with your feet hip width apart and squat down so that your bottom is just off the back of your heels. Touch your fingertips to the floor for balance.

2 Now using both legs, push off and jump into the air. As you land, bend your knees and lower yourself in a controlled way back to the starting position.

3 You will feel this move working your buttocks but you will probably feel your thigh muscles tiring first!

4 Do 4 jumps in a row and then rest in the squat position. Then repeat the 4 jumps. Try to do 5 lots of 4 in total.

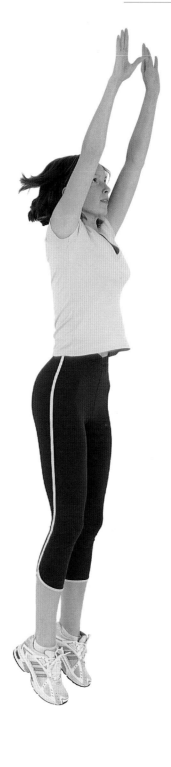

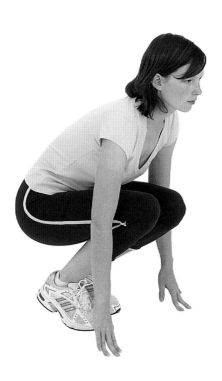

95

groin muscles

To provide all-round balance in the hip area you must also strengthen the groin muscles. Here are some exercises for you to try.

▾ Resistance dynaband pulls

You will feel the work happening in the inner thigh as you pull the leg inwards. Breathe regularly throughout the exercise.

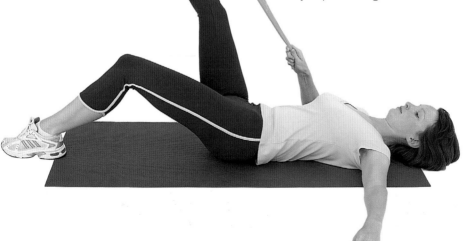

Instructions

1 Lie on the floor with one leg bent with your foot resting on the floor and the other leg raised in the air out to the side. Loop the dynaband around the raised ankle.

2 Now pull the straight leg in towards the centre, trying to resist the dynaband. You will feel the inner thigh muscle tightening as you pull the leg into the mid line.

All the tension should be in your legs as you work the inner thigh/hip muscles.

▶ Ball squeezes

This is what is known as an isometric exercise, i.e. you are working your muscle against something immovable (in this case your other leg). It is important not to hold your breath or tense your upper body as you do the exercise.

Instructions

1 Stand on both feet and place a ball or cushion between your knees.
2 Stand tall with the upper body and squeeze the ball between your knees.

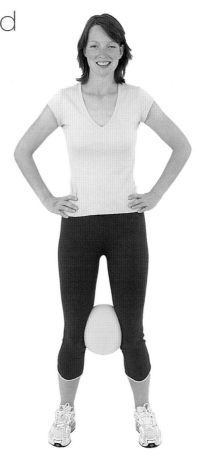

▼ Variation

You can also do this move with a partner.
1 Sit opposite each other with your knees on the outside of your partner's.
2 She will work to squeeze her legs apart and you will use your adductor muscles to squeeze her thighs together.
3 Keep breathing regularly and compete like this for 30 seconds.

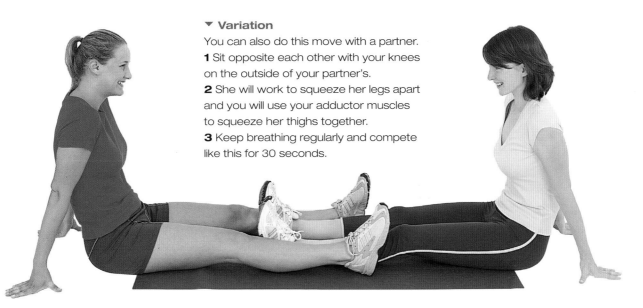

hip flexor muscles

It is not necessary to train the hip flexor muscles heavily as they are kept well trained with activities such as walking, running and climbing stairs. However, it's worth slotting a couple of exercises into your workout routine that work the hip flexors and other key muscles at the same time.

▼ Full sit up

The full sit up is an important exercise as it resembles everyday movement. If you are lying in bed and then you sit upright you are essentially doing a full sit up. The first three-quarters of this exercise will strengthen the abdominals while the last section works the hip flexors.

Instructions

1 Lie on your back with your knees bent. Cross your arms over your chest. If you can get a partner to support your feet, do so. If not, tuck your feet under a chair.

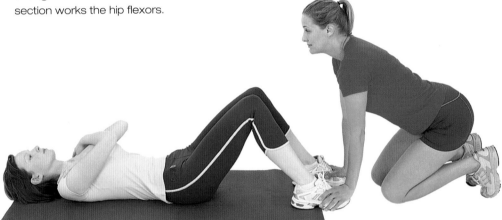

2 Now curl the upper body off the floor and keep curling until your elbows touch your knees.
3 Lower back down with control.
4 Do 20 repetitions but stop if you are too tired to lower yourself back down with sufficient control.

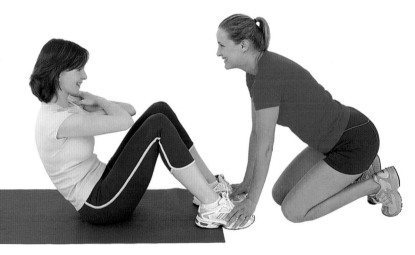

▼ Supine curl ups

Instructions

1 Lie flat on the floor with your arms stretched back behind your head and your legs stretched away from you. Now fix your arms against the floor as if you were hanging onto a bar.

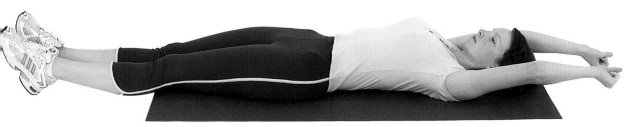

2 Curl your legs up and bring your knees towards your face.
3 Slowly lower your legs back down to full extension on the floor. You will feel the work, from this movement, in both the abdominals and the hip flexors.
4 Repeat this move 10 times

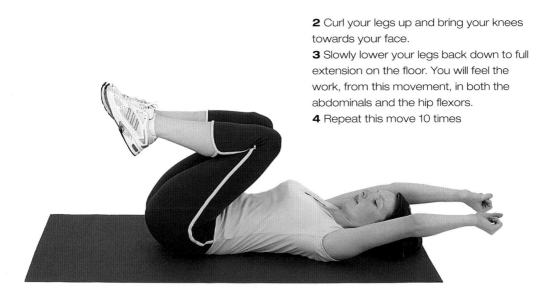

hip stretches

As well as keeping your hip muscles toned, it is important to sustain the mobility and suppleness of this area. The hips, including the joints where the thigh bones fit snugly into the hip sockets, are among the most important joints to keep mobile throughout your life and into old age. As anyone who has needed a hip replacement will tell you, if your hips are out of action so are you! Stretching the muscles around the hips will help keep a full range of movement possible at all times, promoting easy mobility.

Stretch out the front of the hips initially. If you have been doing some of the previous toning exercises or have been sitting down for a long time, you may well feel the urge to stretch them anyway, so here's how to do it.

▶ Leg lifts

Instructions

1 Stand on one leg with one hand holding onto a barre or wall.

2 Take hold of the right leg with the right hand around the ankle. Lift the ankle up behind you as far as you can. Make sure the backward movement takes place at the hip, rather than allowing the back to bend too much.

3 Keep a wide angle at the knee; otherwise you will stretch the quadricep rather than the hip flexors. Hold this stretch for 10–15 seconds and then release.

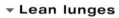

▼ Lean lunges

This stretch works the hip flexors, commonly called the iliopsoas (see page 22).

Instructions

1 Kneel on one knee and place the other foot in front of you on the floor. You may need to place a cushion pad underneath the knee to prevent discomfort.

2 Now press your hips forwards so that you feel a stretch across the front of the hips.

3 Keep pressing the hip forwards into your front knee but don't push the knee beyond the toe, as this will stress the knee.

4 Most stretches of this type, i.e. passive to ensure full range of movement, should be held for 10–15 seconds, then released.

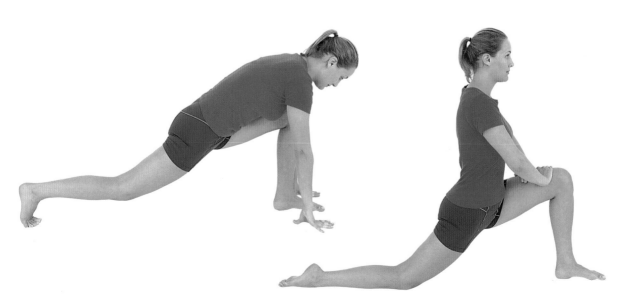

sides of the hips

A s well as stretching the front of the hips, stretch out the sides. Stretching the iliotibial band along the side of the hips and upper thighs is important. If this band gets too tight during training, it can lead to many problems.

▶ Crossed side leans
Instructions

1 Stand with your right foot crossed in front of the other. Push your right hip out to the side slightly.

2 Now lean over, with the upper body to the left side, and hold.

3 Lift up through the body and keep the abdominals tensed for support.

4 Allow your right arm to reach down towards the floor. Hold this stretch for 10–15 seconds and breathe normally all the while. You should feel a stretch down the side of the hip and upper thigh.

If you can hold onto a solid object with your right hand you can angle the body and increase the stretch further.

5 Repeat on the other leg.

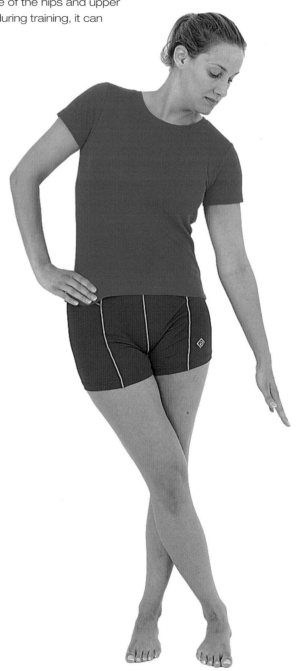

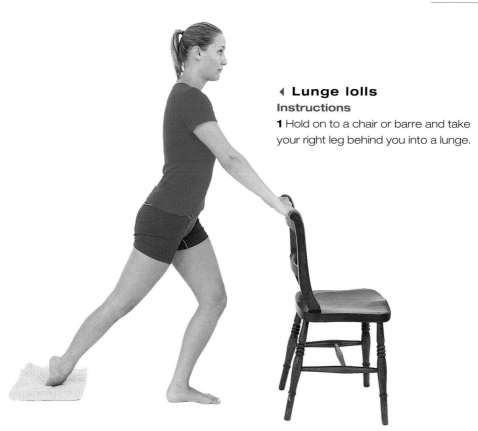

◀ Lunge lolls

Instructions

1 Hold on to a chair or barre and take your right leg behind you into a lunge.

2 Now turn your right foot onto its side. You may need to place a cushion pad underneath the foot for comfort. Lean into the right side of the hip as you bend the left leg a little further.

3 Hold this position for 10–15 seconds and feel the stretch down the right side of the hip and thigh. It is important to keep the tendon band of the iliotibial tract stretched out so that it does not over-tighten.

4 Repeat on the other leg.

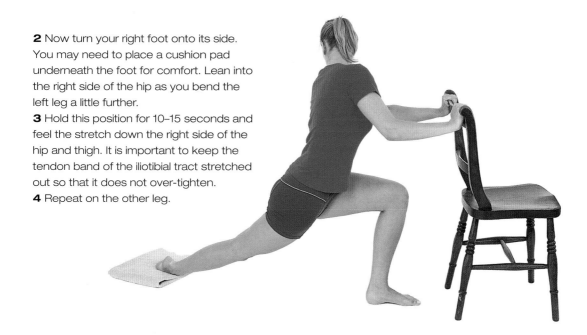

back of the hips

Stretching out the back area of the hips is important for staying balanced and mobile all round. If the buttocks become over-tightened, this can impact on the back. Try the following exercises.

▸ Sit sos
Instructions

1 Sit with one leg straight out in front of you. Pull the other leg in towards you with both hands.

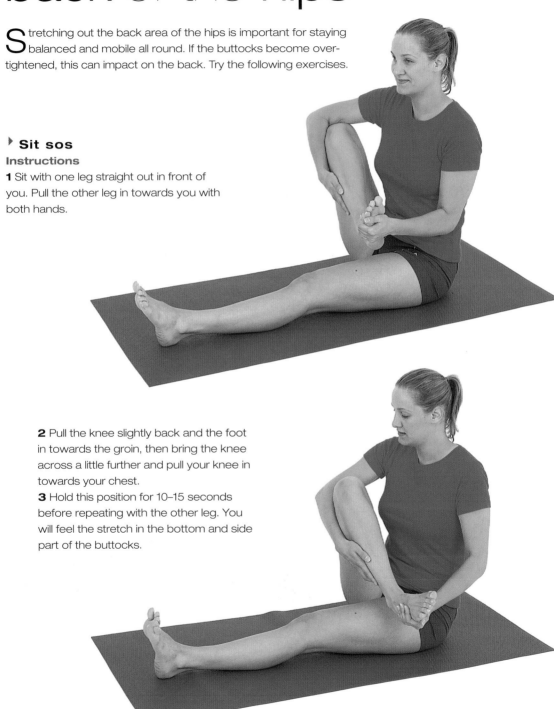

2 Pull the knee slightly back and the foot in towards the groin, then bring the knee across a little further and pull your knee in towards your chest.
3 Hold this position for 10–15 seconds before repeating with the other leg. You will feel the stretch in the bottom and side part of the buttocks.

▼ 'L' crosses

Instructions

1 Lie on the floor with one leg bent and the other straight. Use the opposite hand from your bent leg to reach down and take hold of your knee.

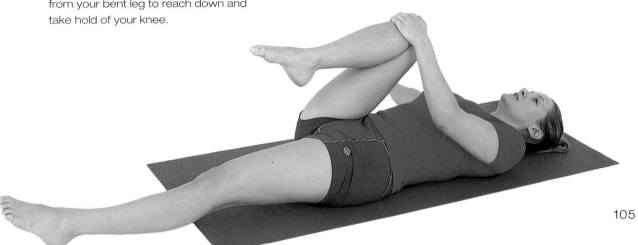

2 Gently pull your knee across your body and hold when you feel the stretch down the side of your hip, across the buttock and down the side of the thigh. However, depending on how tight you are, you may feel this stretch in some areas and not others. If your back is quite tight, you may feel some tension in the lower back as you twist. As long as this is not uncomfortable, this position is fine.

3 Hold for 10–15 seconds and then return your leg to the floor. Repeat with the other leg coming across.

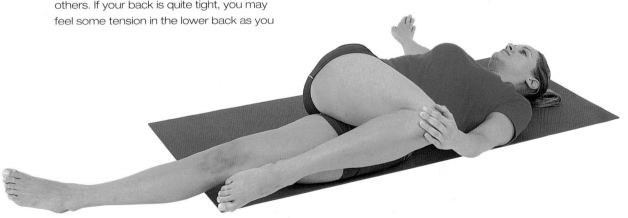

part 7

thigh exercises

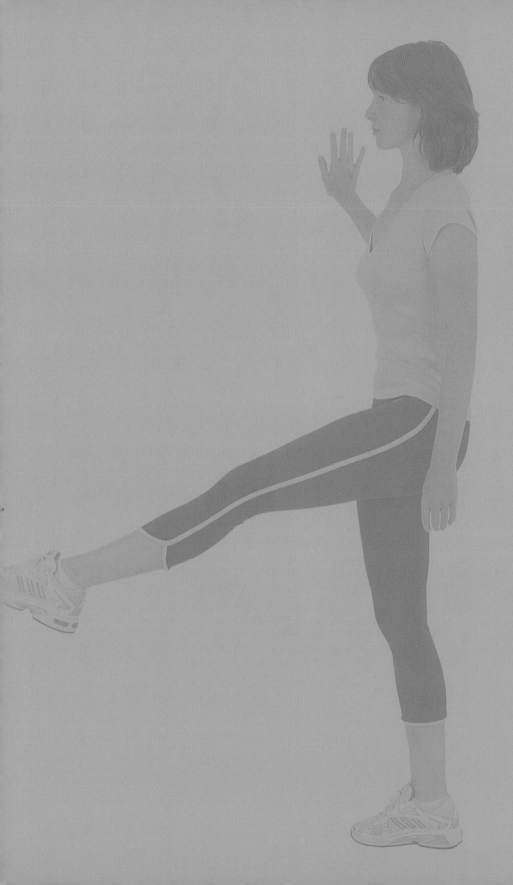

thigh toners

Some of the best exercises for toning the thighs are those in which both your knees are bending and pushing the weight of your body upwards. Try out the following simple moves to feel the burn!

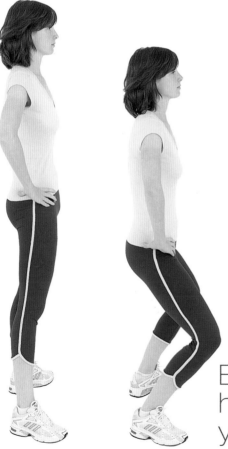

◀ Wide plies

You will feel the stretch on the inner thighs and the work on the outer thighs if you are lowering yourself slowly enough.

Instructions

1 Stand with your feet a width and a half of your shoulders, turning your feet out slightly.
2 With the plie move, you bend the knees slowly, as you do with the squat, but taking your bottom (and hips) directly down. Don't push your backside out to the back as you do with a squat. The consequence of this is that it engages the inner and outer thigh muscles more and works the mobility of the hip joints. Place your hands on your hips to guide them where to go!
3 Perform 10 slow moves up and down, then shake out your legs and repeat.

Be tough and aim those hips down directly below you, even if it hurts!

▼ Squats

The squat is a classic move that most people know but it is still worth doing regularly to keep your thighs strong.

Instructions

1 Stand with your feet hip width apart and your abdominals pulled up.

2 Lower yourself by bending your legs and pushing your bottom out behind you. Keep your abdominals tight so that your back does not arch. Bend your knees until you feel the weight over your heels. Your upper body should be in a straight line from your shoulders to your hips.

3 As you come up again, remember to keep the abdominals and the pelvic floor muscles tense and straighten your legs.
4 Perform 10 slow and controlled moves, then shake out your legs and repeat.

109

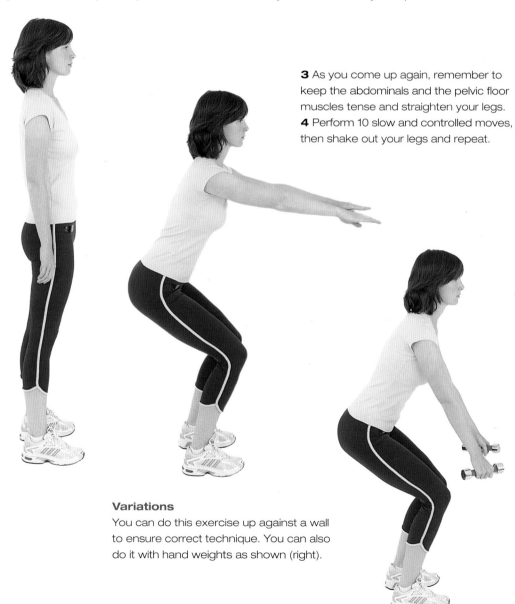

Variations

You can do this exercise up against a wall to ensure correct technique. You can also do it with hand weights as shown (right).

ballet work

One of the reasons why ballet dancers have such strong-looking legs is that they do an enormous amount of work on one leg. Try one of their moves to get a feel of how hard it is!

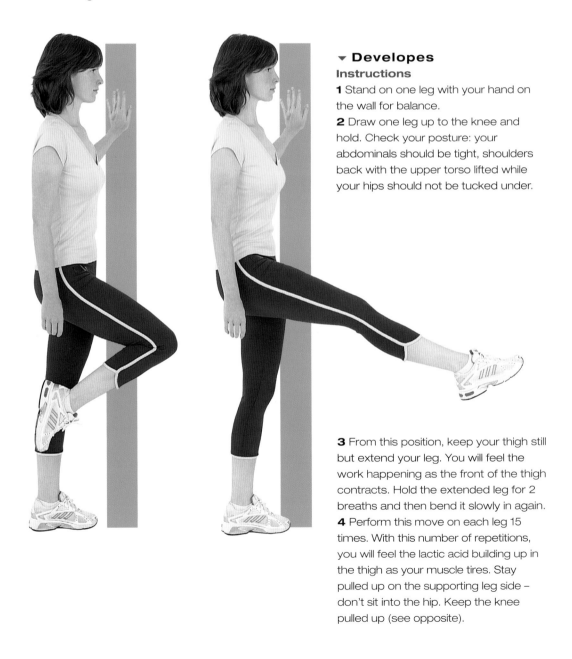

▼ Developes
Instructions

1 Stand on one leg with your hand on the wall for balance.
2 Draw one leg up to the knee and hold. Check your posture: your abdominals should be tight, shoulders back with the upper torso lifted while your hips should not be tucked under.

3 From this position, keep your thigh still but extend your leg. You will feel the work happening as the front of the thigh contracts. Hold the extended leg for 2 breaths and then bend it slowly in again.
4 Perform this move on each leg 15 times. With this number of repetitions, you will feel the lactic acid building up in the thigh as your muscle tires. Stay pulled up on the supporting leg side – don't sit into the hip. Keep the knee pulled up (see opposite).

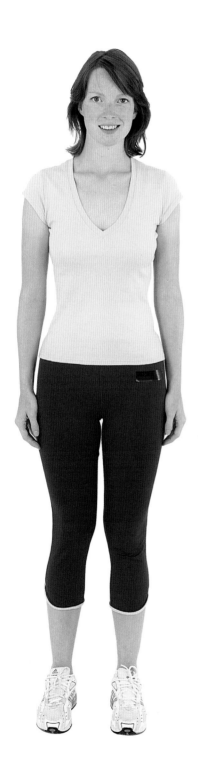

◀ Static knee contractions

One of the most important moves for keeping the legs toned is a simple contraction that can be done anywhere; it should be used whenever you stand straight. The static knee contraction is simply the act of pulling up the knee cap on the leg.

Instructions

1 Stand up straight and pull up the knee caps of both legs – this involves tensing the thighs. Maintain this movement as you stand with both legs straight or when you stand on one leg. This not only keeps the thighs tensed but also ensures there is no pushing back at the back of the knee – hyper-extension – which is potentially dangerous to the joint.

2 Whenever you stand on one leg, as in the exercise opposite, try to keep the static contraction of the knees in place. Although this takes effort, it builds heat, muscle tone and correct posture.

111

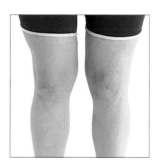

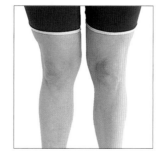

outer thighs

The following exercises will work the important outer thigh area and will really tone up these muscles, making your thighs look firmer and trimmer.

▼ Classic abductor lifts

Instructions

1 Lie on your side, propped up on one elbow. Make sure your hips are stacked one on top of the other, your knees bent at right angles and your abdominals are tight. Place one hand on the floor in front of you to prevent you falling forwards.

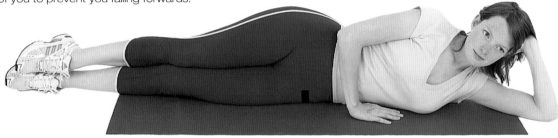

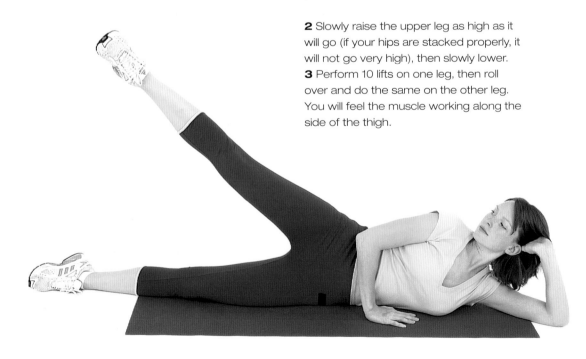

2 Slowly raise the upper leg as high as it will go (if your hips are stacked properly, it will not go very high), then slowly lower.
3 Perform 10 lifts on one leg, then roll over and do the same on the other leg. You will feel the muscle working along the side of the thigh.

▼ Ball flies

This is another static contraction move, i.e. when there is no movement other than the muscle contracting, and it will work the outer thigh rotator muscles. You will feel the work on the side of the thigh almost into the buttocks.

Instructions

1 Lie on your front and place a ball or cushion between your feet.

When you do an isometric or static contraction move, keep breathing naturally.

113

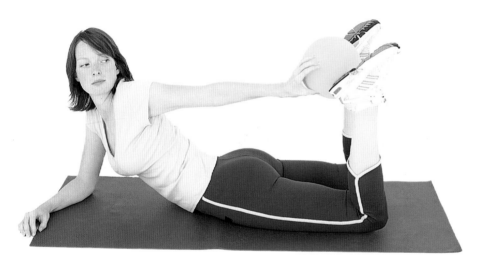

2 Bend your knees and hold the position. From here, squeeze the ball with both feet as if you are trying to push your feet together.
3 Hold the squeeze for 30 seconds, then rest and repeat.

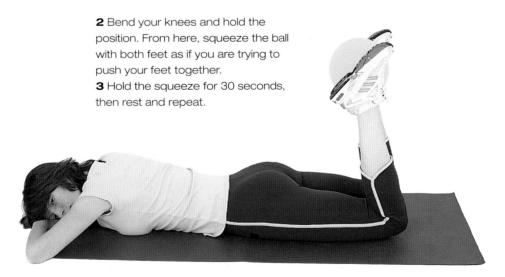

inner thigh muscles

The muscles on the inner thighs need working too. Squeezing the legs together (or into the mid line) works these muscles. Try the following exercises.

▼ Attitude lifts

The aim here is to turn the thigh outwards and drop the knee slightly, lifting the side of the foot towards the ceiling.

Instructions

1 Stand on one foot with the other leg pulled up (see the static knee contraction exercise on page 111).

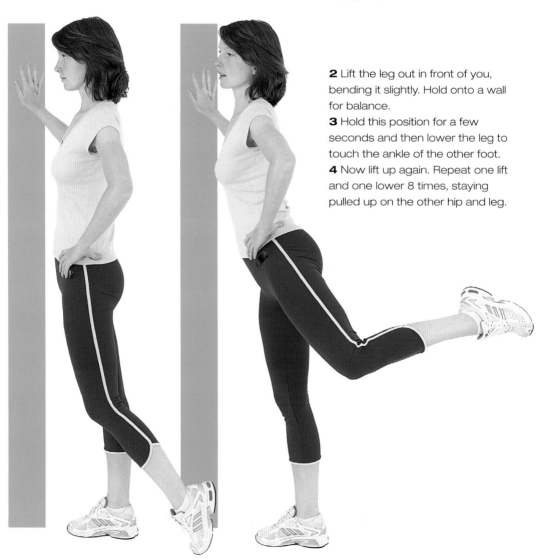

2 Lift the leg out in front of you, bending it slightly. Hold onto a wall for balance.
3 Hold this position for a few seconds and then lower the leg to touch the ankle of the other foot.
4 Now lift up again. Repeat one lift and one lower 8 times, staying pulled up on the other hip and leg.

▼ Hamstring stresses

It is not necessary to do huge amounts of work on the back of the thigh but one exercise is a good idea to keep the muscle groups balanced.

Instructions

1 Lie down on your front and press your hips firmly into the floor. Now extend your feet, pointing your toes, and bring your heels together.

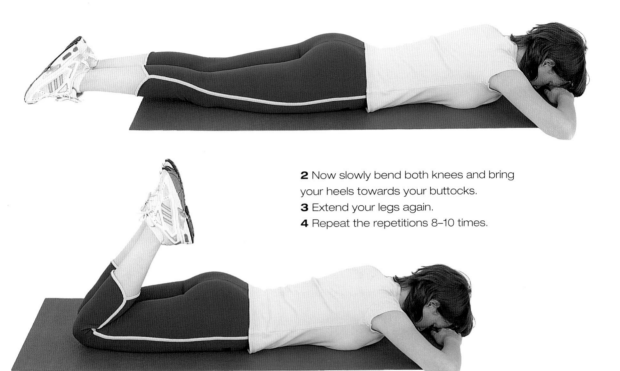

2 Now slowly bend both knees and bring your heels towards your buttocks.
3 Extend your legs again.
4 Repeat the repetitions 8–10 times.

115

Variations

This exercise will feel relatively easy but you can increase the intensity by weighting your legs down with some ankle weights, or you can get a partner to resist your legs as you bring them in.

thigh stretches

Regular mobility and stretching work on the legs will make you more supple and aid movement as well as keeping the muscles long and lean. The hamstrings at the back of the leg are used in all forward motion and can get particularly tight. If they tighten too much, they can affect the lower back, so stretching them out is a wise move.

▼ 'L' sits

Instructions

1 Sit on the floor with one leg straight and the other leg bent, with your foot pressed into the inner thigh.
2 Sit up tall, pull in on your abdominals and reach forwards as far as you can.
3 If you can, take hold of your foot and pull yourself gently towards your knee.
4 Hold this position for 10–15 seconds and then slowly release.

Variations

If you can't reach your foot, don't worry; just place your hands on either side of your leg and lean forwards as far as you can. Try to breathe evenly throughout.

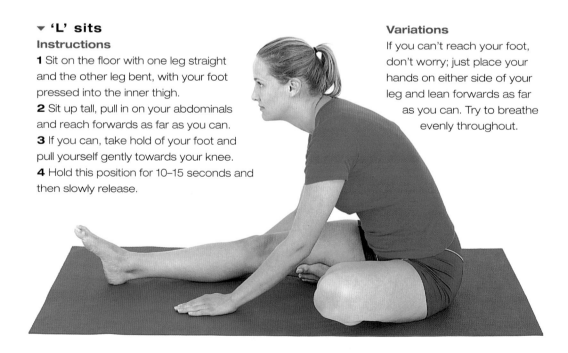

▶ Yoga flexes

This useful hamstring stretch has been adapted from yoga.

Instructions

1 Lie on your back and lift one leg up towards you. If possible, the leg should be straight; if not, keep the knee bent.

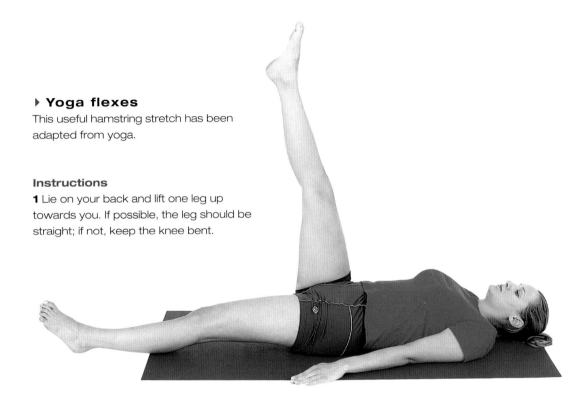

2 Hook your fingers around the toes of the raised leg, then try to pull (very gently and slowly) the leg towards your head.
3 Once you have lifted the leg as far as is mildly uncomfortable, hold this position for 10–15 seconds, then release the leg. If your knee is bent, this is fine and you will still feel the stretch on the back of your thigh as you hold the position.

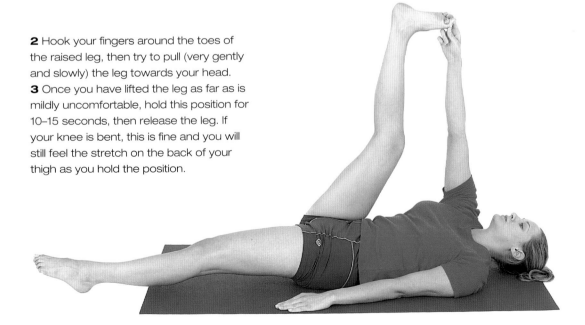

inner thigh muscles

Stretching the inner thigh muscles is just as important as keeping the hamstrings flexible. If both sets of muscles are pliable, then you will have the best movement advantage!

▶ 1st sits
Instructions

1 Sit with your feet together and knees open. Hold onto your ankles and press the knees down towards the floor as far as you can.

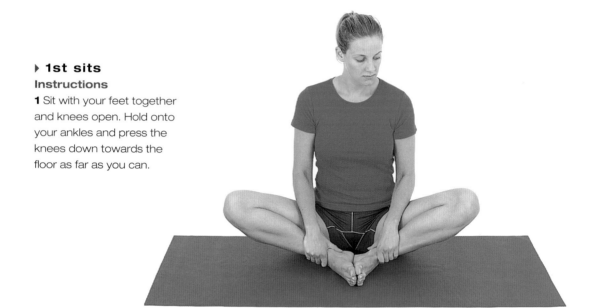

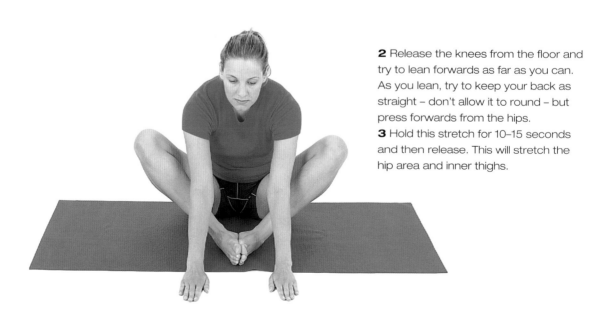

2 Release the knees from the floor and try to lean forwards as far as you can. As you lean, try to keep your back as straight – don't allow it to round – but press forwards from the hips.
3 Hold this stretch for 10–15 seconds and then release. This will stretch the hip area and inner thighs.

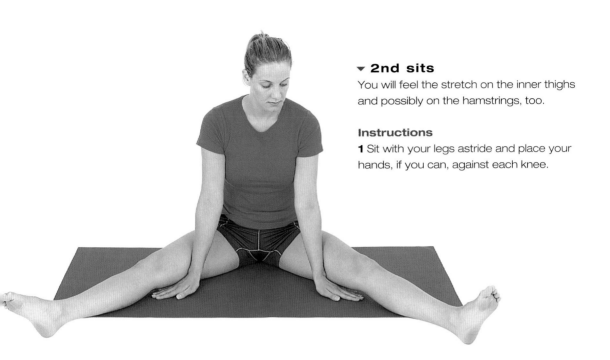

▼ 2nd sits

You will feel the stretch on the inner thighs and possibly on the hamstrings, too.

Instructions

1 Sit with your legs astride and place your hands, if you can, against each knee.

2 Slowly try to lean forwards as far as you can. Hold this position for 10–15 seconds and then release the stretch.
3 If you can't reach to get your hands in this position, don't worry. Just reach the hands slowly forwards. The purpose of placing your hands in this position is to keep your knees back (not rolling in) as you lean forwards.

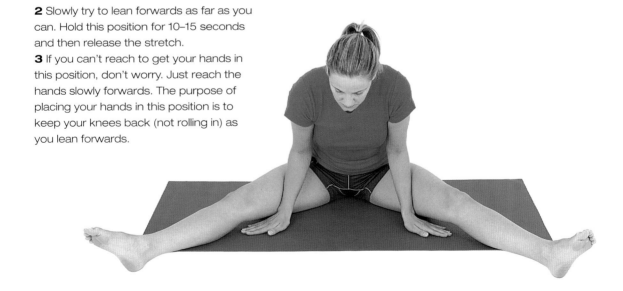

front of the thigh muscles

The muscles at the front of the thigh (see page 23) also need to be kept long and lean so practise the following stretches for this important area.

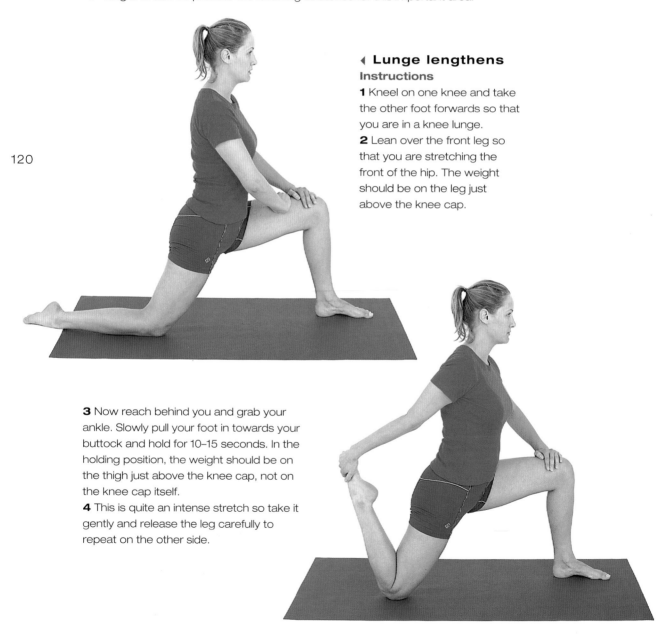

◀ Lunge lengthens
Instructions

1 Kneel on one knee and take the other foot forwards so that you are in a knee lunge.
2 Lean over the front leg so that you are stretching the front of the hip. The weight should be on the leg just above the knee cap.

3 Now reach behind you and grab your ankle. Slowly pull your foot in towards your buttock and hold for 10–15 seconds. In the holding position, the weight should be on the thigh just above the knee cap, not on the knee cap itself.
4 This is quite an intense stretch so take it gently and release the leg carefully to repeat on the other side.

▼ Lying lengthens

Instructions

1 Lie on your front, resting on your elbows. Reach behind with one hand and grab your foot.

2 Draw the foot gently in towards the buttock. You will feel quite a stretch on the front of the thigh.

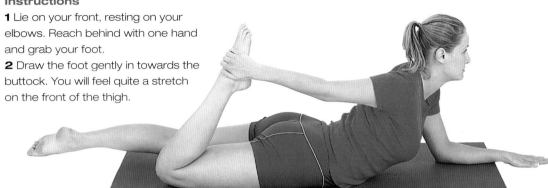

3 If this stretch feels relatively gentle, straighten your supporting arm so that your upper body is raised up higher. This will increase the stretch on the thigh.

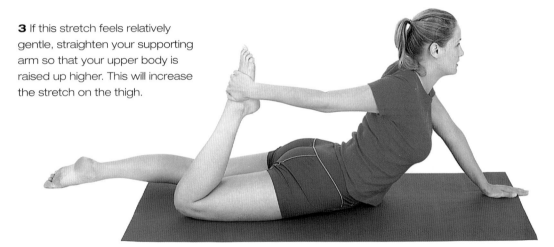

4 Now perform the same action with your leg, pulling the foot in to the buttock. This should feel a much more intense stretch.

5 Hold for 10–15 seconds, then release and repeat on the other leg.

Note: Do not do this last part if you have any problems with your knees.

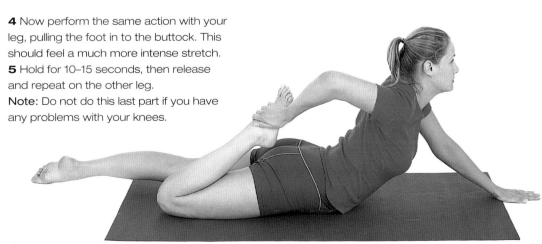

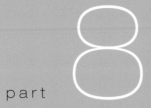

part 8

122

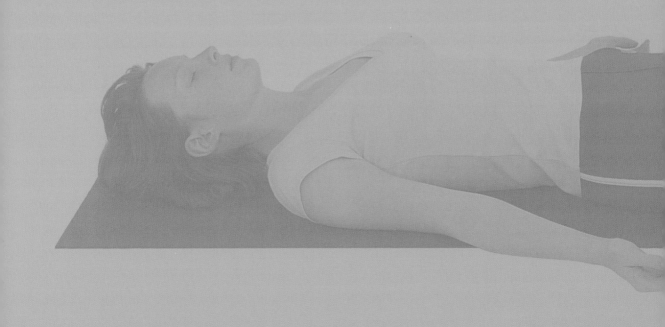

cool
down

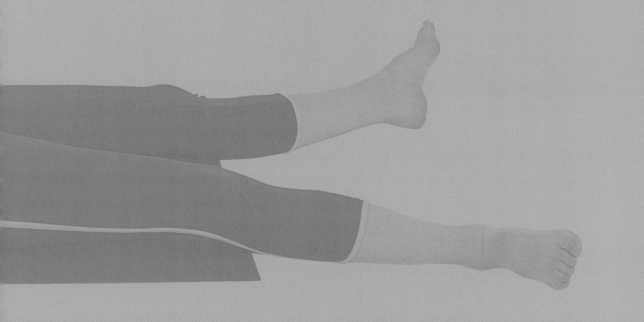

cooling down

When you've done a hard workout, even if it is just 10 minutes, your body needs time at the end to readjust. Yoga practice suggests a prone position for at least 10 minutes after the activity just to let the body realign. Try these different approaches and see which cool down suits you best.

▼ Prone check

Instructions

1 After you have completed your hip and thigh workout, lie on the floor flat on your back and just breathe.

2 Allow the body to sink into the floor, concentrating on feeling the muscles release. This may take a couple of seconds. Do not allow yourself to drift off mentally but keep focused on your body. After some moments you should start to notice that suddenly one muscle seems to be letting go a little and that your limb is falling into the floor. Try to register this happening throughout your body. Register the different feelings in your body. You may feel some discomfort as you feel the muscles let go, after working hard.

3 Stay in this position for about 5–8 minutes until all the discomfort has disappeared and your body has completely relaxed into the floor.

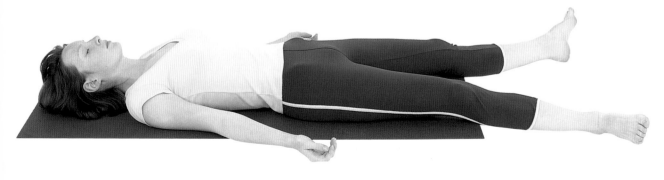

▼ Relaxation stretch

Stretching can be used in several ways.
Many stretches return the muscles to
pre-exercise length at the end of a
workout. Some extend their range of
flexibility while others are great for
relaxation. To stretch for relaxation,
you have to be in a position that feels
comfortable in order to stay there
for longer and to stretch certain
muscles at the same time.

Instructions

1 Lie on the floor and bring both knees
into your chest. Wrap your arms across
your knees and hold. Breathe evenly in
this position.

125

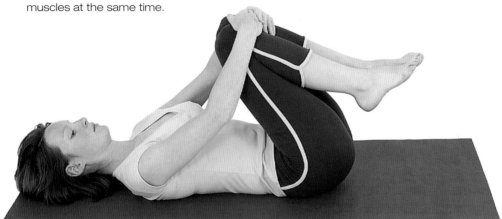

2 Now gently add some simple pressure.
Breathe in. As you breathe out, gently hug
your knees in tighter to your chest. Let
the pressure relax as you breathe in
again. You will find this stretch feels really
good at the back of the hips because it
releases and stretches the lower back.
3 Stay in this position for as long as it
feels good, usually about 10–12 breaths.

▼ Dance cool down

After a particularly hard session it is best not to stop dead in your tracks and fall to the floor! Sometimes you need to allow your pulse to return to normal as you do some gentle moves to slow down.

Instructions

1 If you are really hot, march on the spot.
2 Then take two steps to one side and two steps to the other.
3 Now perform some active stretches. Stand on one leg and kick with the other. Do 4 kicks on each leg.

4 March again and finally reach up with both hands as high as you can, stretching right through your body, then drop your hands down.
5 Repeat this whole sequence, getting progressively slower and less energetic with each move.

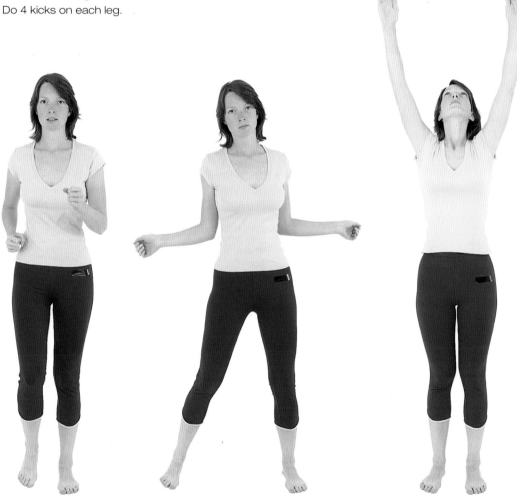

Rehydrate!

Too many people forget to eat and drink after a major workout! Your body needs to refuel in order to have the energy to keep going. Not only this, but if you have worked your muscles hard you may need to eat some complex carbohydrates within two hours of a tough muscle session to provide the calories your body needs to build new muscle. If you forget to drink, you can land yourself with a lot of problems. Feelings of tiredness or headaches can be brought on by dehydration. Although it sounds extreme, low-level dehydration can occur frequently without people even being aware of it. If you exercise regularly, you will sweat regularly so it important to drink water after every workout. Aim to drink 225 ml (8 fl oz) every hour on the days you exercise.

index